Intestinal Obstructions

Edited by Dmitry Victorovich Garbuzenko

Published in London, United Kingdom

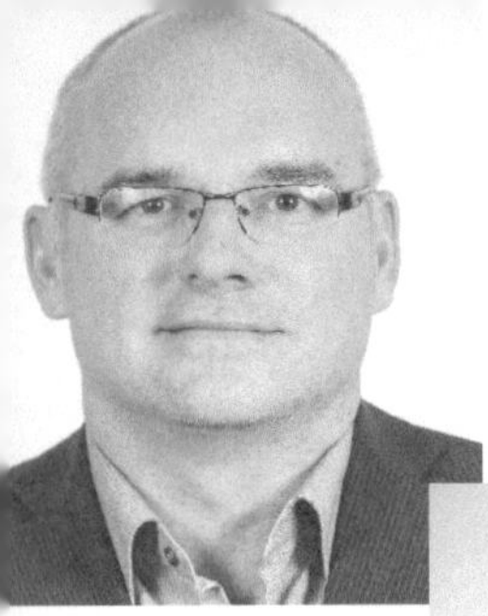
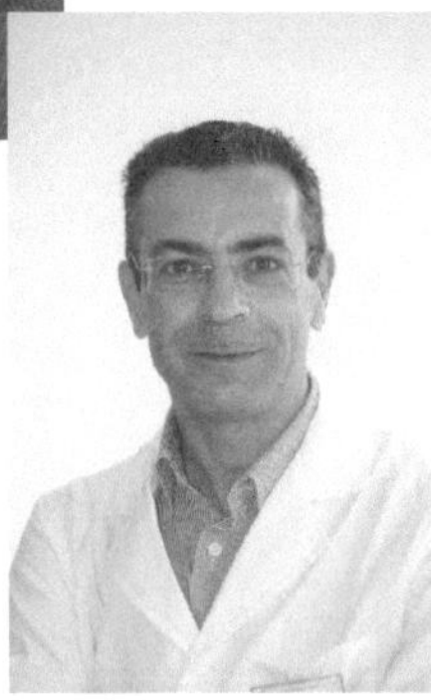
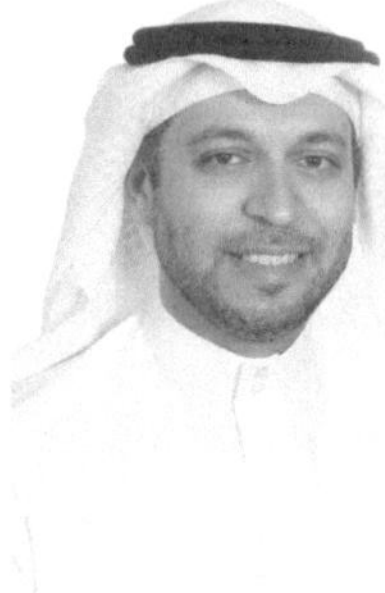
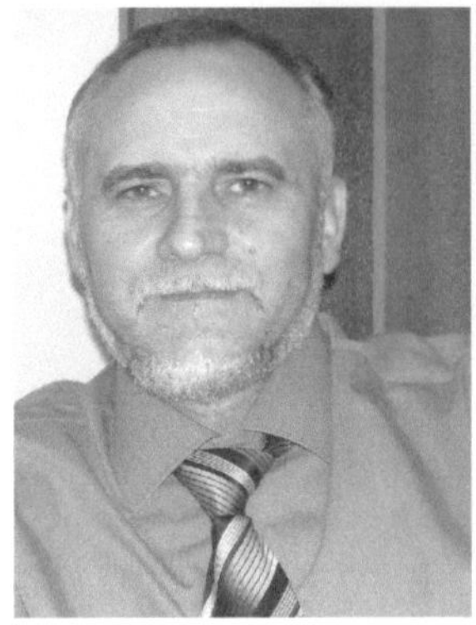
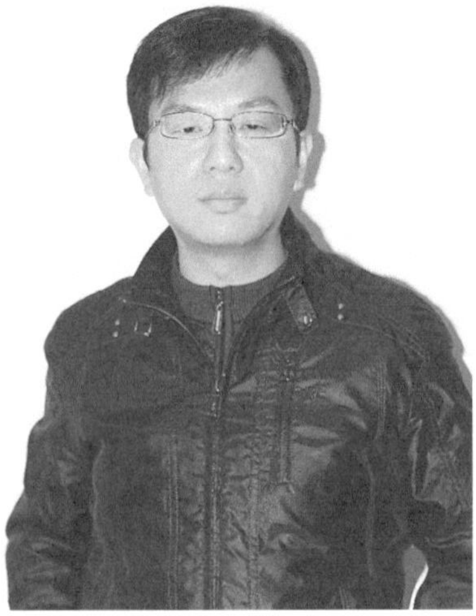
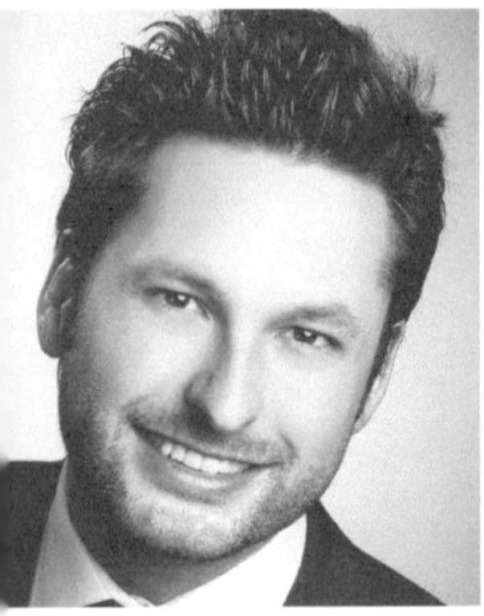
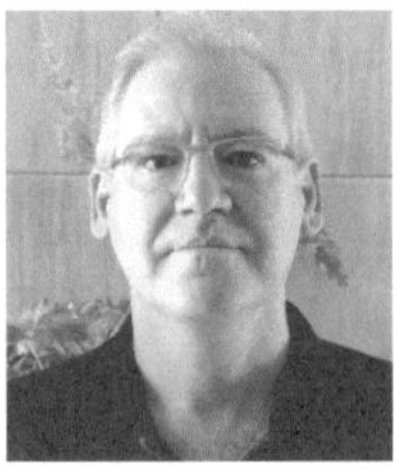

IntechOpen

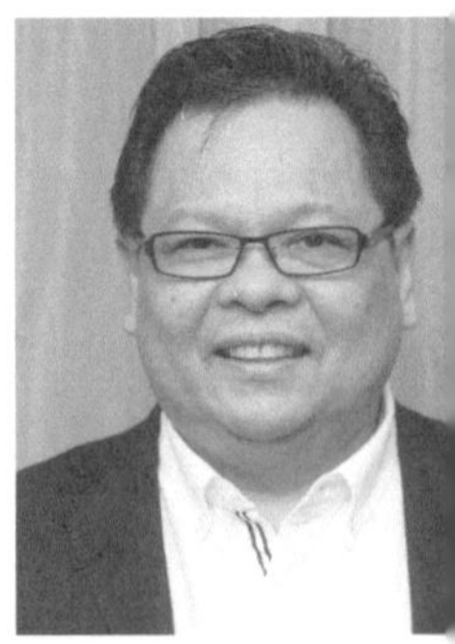
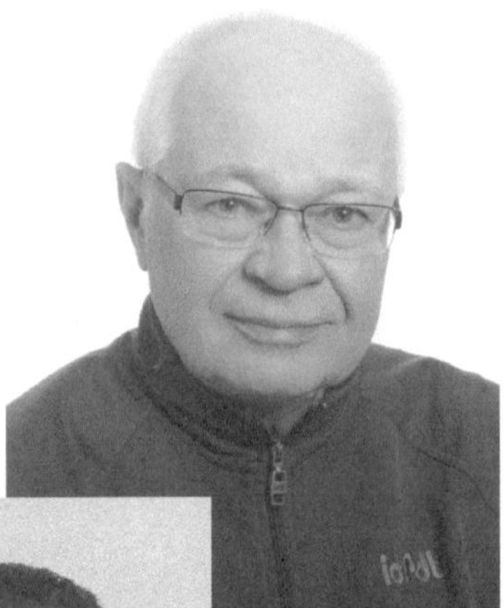
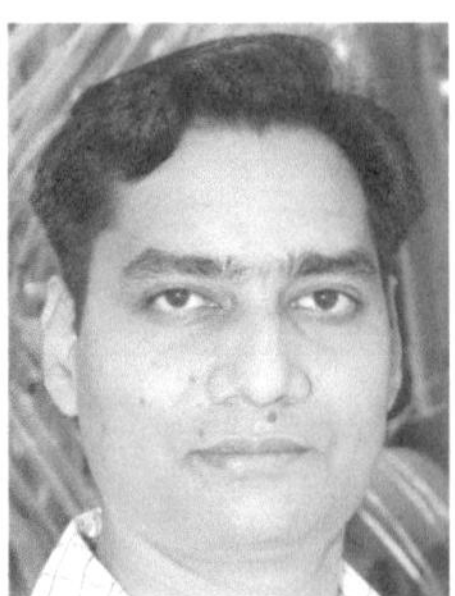
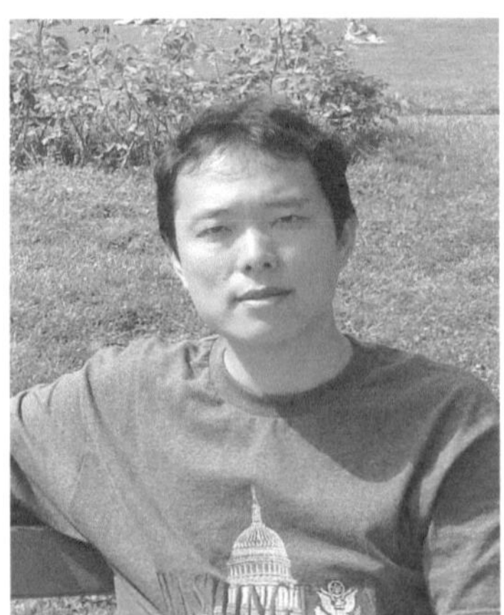
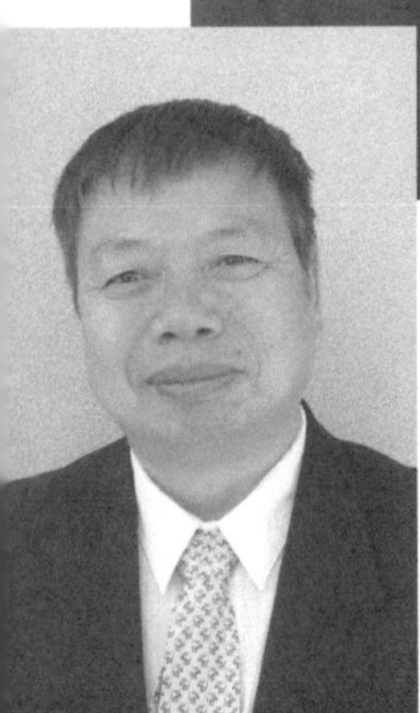
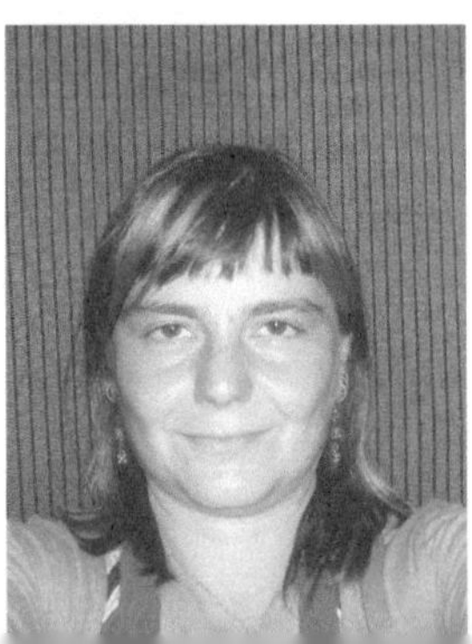

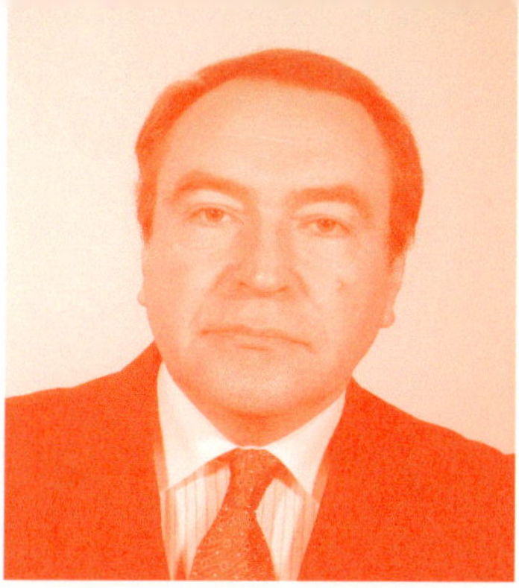
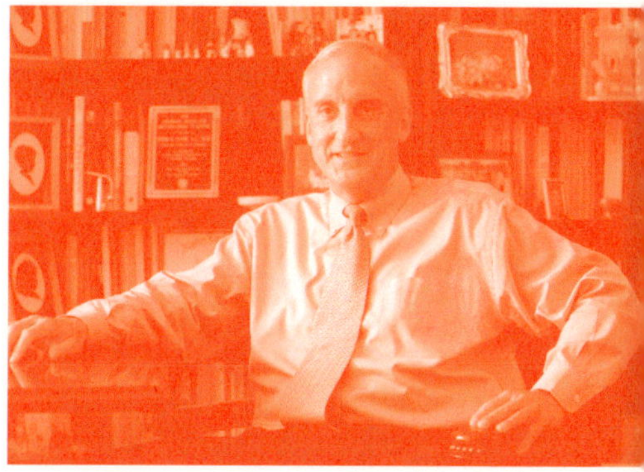
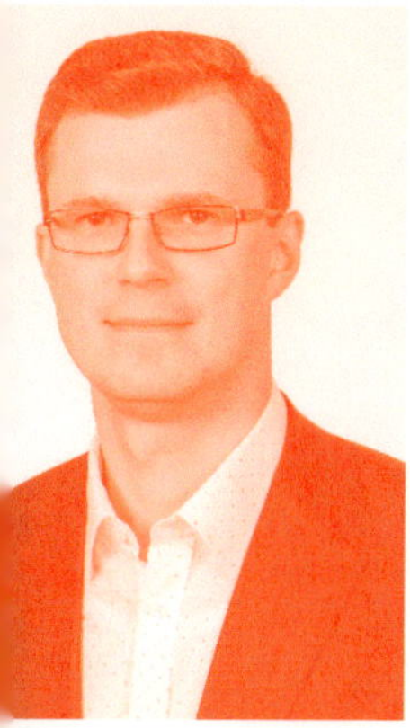
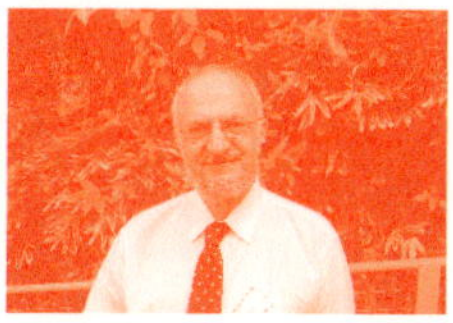
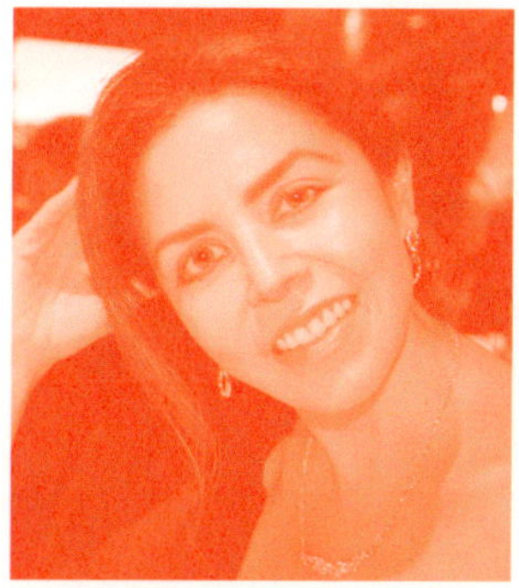

Supporting open minds since 2005

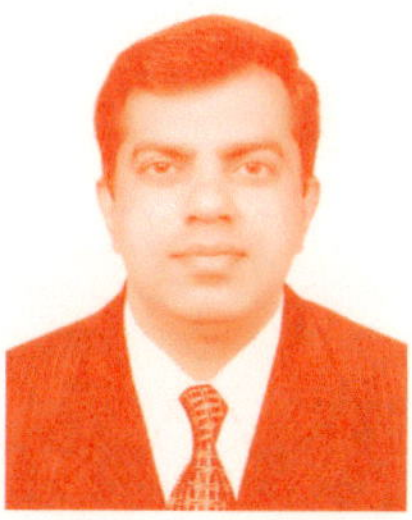
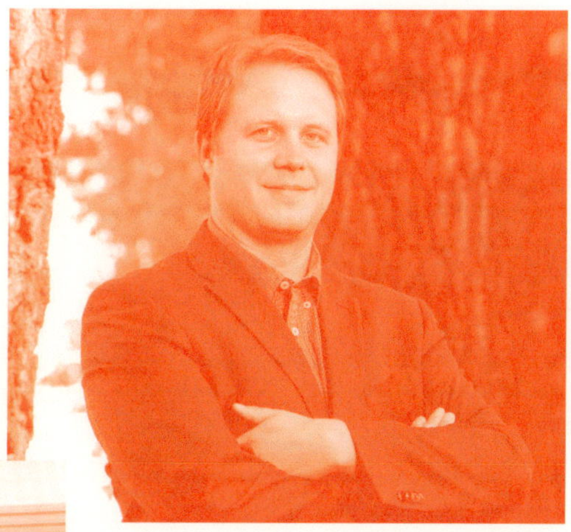
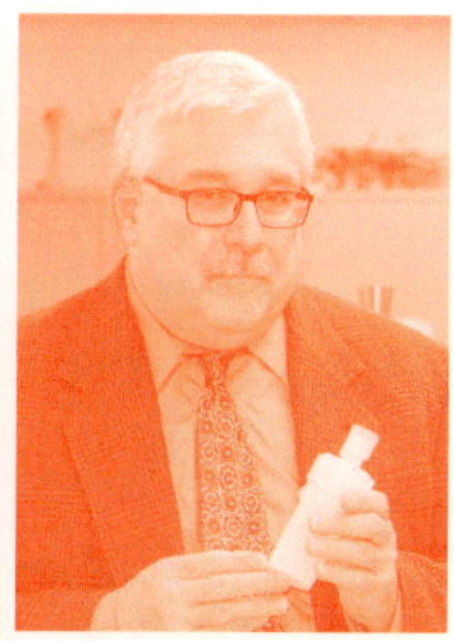
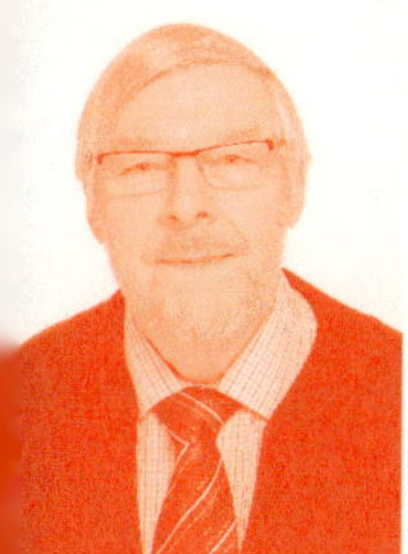
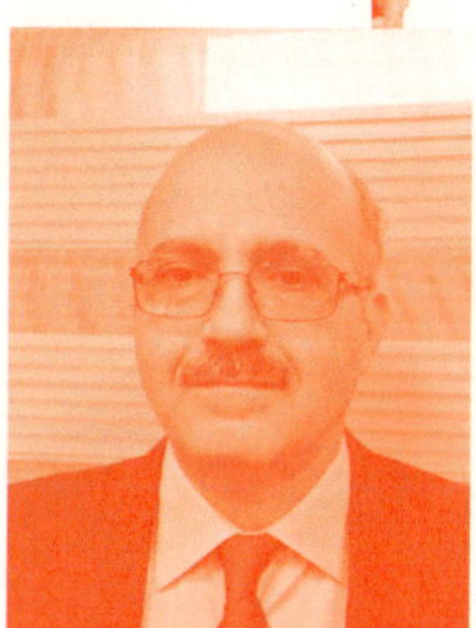
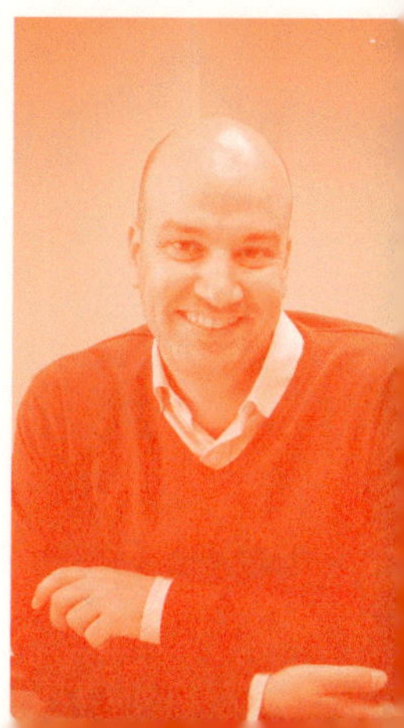
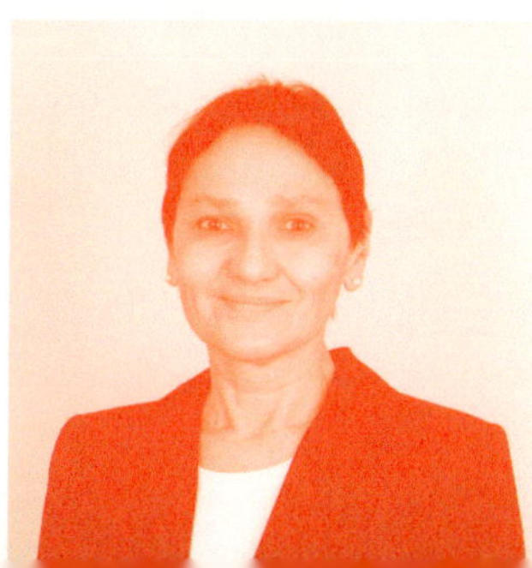

Intestinal Obstructions
http://dx.doi.org/10.5772/intechopen.89823
Edited by Dmitry Victorovich Garbuzenko

Contributors
Giovanni Petracca, Francesco Zappia, Fabrizio Silvaggio, Paul K. Okeny, Víctor Hugo García Orozco, Pepijn Krielen, Martijn W. J Stommel, Richard P. G. Ten Broek, Harry Van Goor, Jessica Taylor, Devin Clegg, Dmitry Victorovich Garbuzenko

First published in London, United Kingdom, 2021 by IntechOpen
IntechOpen is the global imprint of INTECHOPEN LIMITED, registered in England and Wales, registration number: 11086078, 5 Princes Gate Court, London, SW7 2QJ, United Kingdom
Printed in Croatia

British Library Cataloguing-in-Publication Data
A catalogue record for this book is available from the British Library

Additional hard and PDF copies can be obtained from orders@intechopen.com

Intestinal Obstructions
Edited by Dmitry Victorovich Garbuzenko
p. cm.
Print ISBN 978-1-78985-129-8
Online ISBN 978-1-78985-130-4
eBook (PDF) ISBN 978-1-83962-587-9

Meet the editor

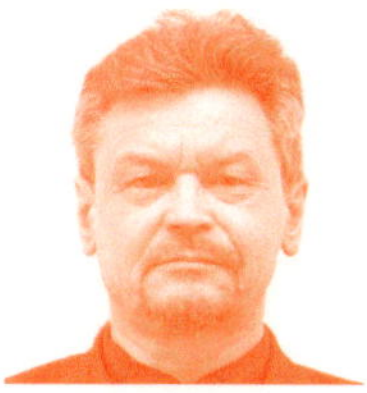

Dmitry Victorovich Garbuzenko graduated from Chelyabinsk State Medical Institute in 1985. From 1985 to 1987, he was a clinical intern. From 1987 to 1990, he was a post-graduate student of the Hospital Surgery Department in Chelyabinsk State Medical Academy. He obtained his Ph.D. in 1991. He was an assistant professor of the Department of Hospital Surgery from 1991 to 1996. Since 1996, he has served as an assistant professor, an associate professor (2003), and a full professor (2006) in the Department of Faculty Surgery, South Ural State Medical University. He obtained his DMedSc in 2008. Dr. Garbuzenko is a member of the Russian Society of Surgeons. His practical activities associate with emergency abdominal surgery. He is the author of nearly 180 publications.

Contents

Preface

A group of pathological conditions characterized by the impaired passage of contents from the stomach to the rectum as well as the intestinal obstruction is associated with a very severe course, difficulty in diagnosis, and an unfavorable outcome. Mechanical intestinal obstruction is a current problem of emergency abdominal surgery. The frequency of intestinal obstruction is about 5 cases per 100,000, accounting for 3% to 5% of admissions to emergency surgical hospitals. Among all types of obstruction, small bowel obstruction predominates, which is distinguished by complex clinical manifestations and a poor prognosis. As a rule, it occurs due to adhesions after previous operations. However, there are also rarer causes, for example, gallstones, bezoars, and others. Large bowel obstruction, being one of the most common and dangerous complications of colon cancer, is observed in 15% to 75% of cases. Intestinal strangulation, caused by volvulus or incarceration, is the most insidious due to the rapid onset of ischemia and necrosis of the intestine and always requires urgent surgical intervention. Intestinal intussusception usually occurs in young children and, with timely diagnosis, can be successfully eliminated by conservative or endoscopic methods. Written by an international team of highly qualified specialists, this book will be of interest to anyone engaged in emergency abdominal surgery.

Dmitry Victorovich Garbuzenko
Professor,
Department of Faculty Surgery,
South Ural State Medical University,
Chelyabinsk, Russia

Chapter 1

Introductory Chapter: Nuances of Surgical Technique for the Treatment of Adhesive Small Bowel Obstruction

Dmitry Garbuzenko

1. Introduction

Adhesive small bowel obstruction is one of the most formidable urgent surgical diseases of the abdominal organs [1]. Surgeons that encounter this disease are well aware of how insidious it is and how difficult it is to treat this pathology. Adhesive small bowel obstruction may often be successfully resolved conservatively. However, if conservative treatment is not effective within 72 h, and if there are signs of peritonitis, strangulation, or bowel ischemia, surgery is necessary [2]. Very often, a surgeon on call decides on the necessity of surgery. This surgeon might not have a lot of experience, but has to deal with the disease face-to-face. However, even experienced specialists may run into significant difficulties during such surgical interventions [3]. The only way to disengage from such a situation with honor is to strictly follow tactics and techniques developed by doctors involved in emergency abdominal surgery. In this chapter, I would like to share the nuances of performing surgery in patients with acute adhesive small bowel obstruction, based on more than 35-year experience of night shifts in an urgent surgical clinic.

2. Surgical access

Despite the achievements of laparoscopic surgery, in most cases of adhesive small bowel obstruction, surgery is performed via a wide incision of the anterior abdominal wall. The optimal surgical approach is midline laparotomy, which, if necessary, is extended up to the umbilicus or down to the pubic symphysis. If the patient has previously undergone midline laparotomy, it is expedient to start surgery with an incision upper or lower the scar. In any case, the scar, encapsulated non-absorbable sutures, and granulation tissue are excised, and the incision is treated with an antiseptic solution.

The parietal peritoneum in the area of the postoperative scar of the anterior abdominal wall always has gross adhesions with aponeurosis forming the *linea alba*. Moreover, as a rule, internal organs are fixed to the *linea alba* by adhesions. Therefore, the peritoneum should be lifted with tweezers and opened very carefully, since the dilated bowel loops may be easily damaged. It is better to keep the surgical site dry for a better view but achieve it without electrocauterization. When a small penetration into the abdominal cavity is achieved, the available area of the peritoneal cavity is carefully examined with a finger. Next, the abdominal wall is lifted with

IntechOpen

a Farabeuf retractor or Maikulicz clamp applied to the aponeurosis edge, and the adhered organs are bluntly and sharply dissected; so, the aponeurosis and parietal peritoneum are prepared for the subsequent extension of the incision. When the abdominal cavity is opened, the dilated loops of the small bowel tend to slip out and should be kept with gauze pads moistened in an antiseptic solution. The gauze pads should be fixed, so as not to accidentally leave them in the peritoneal cavity.

3. Examination of the abdominal cavity

Sometimes the cause of intestinal obstruction is detected immediately, but more often an examination of the abdominal cavity is required. First of all, palpation should be performed. If it yields no result, the intestine should be moved to the left to try to isolate and examine the cecum. Obviously, the cecum is constricted in small bowel obstruction and dilated in large bowel obstruction. When the level of intestinal obstruction is determined, the next step is to search for an obstacle. To identify adhesions that obstructed the small bowel, it is necessary to examine it in the oral direction, starting from the cecum. The site of obstruction is where the constricted small bowel becomes dilated.

Such manipulations are possible only if the bowel is moderately dilated and adhesions are mild. Otherwise, a surgeon has to sort through the intestinal loops sequentially, which is difficult to do without preliminary nasointestinal intubation.

4. Technique of adhesiolysis

Adhesiolysis is started when the site of obstruction is found. The dissection of "loose" adhesions, which are more common in early adhesive bowel obstruction, is not technically difficult. Such adhesions can be destroyed with a finger, but undue force should not be exerted as it may lead to damage to the serous layer of the intestine. Otherwise, adhesions may be cut with scissors. In the latter case, scissors are used in a reverse manner. The tips of closed scissors are inserted between the adhered organs and then opened to separate them. This helps to find the "layer" between the bowel loops fixed to each other.

The greatest technical difficulties arise when the long portions of bowel loops are intimately fixed to each other and/or to the parietal peritoneum. The resulting single conglomerate is sometimes so dense that it is almost impossible to identify the borderline between the organs. In such cases, the safest way to separate the intestine is to excise it with the adjacent peritoneum.

To eliminate dense planar intestinal adhesions, space is created in the place of their least severity in the direction of the posterior abdominal wall. The index finger of the right hand is introduced into this space and the adhesions are separated along the posterior surface of the intestinal conglomerate by pendulum-like movements and without excessive force. As a rule, their density in this area is not so pronounced, so there is a chance to partially release the intestinal loops located there. After reaching some mobility, the bowel loops are rotated anteriorly, and the dissection of adhesions is completed. If it is not possible to separate the obstruction-causing conglomerate of the bowel loops, then, in the absence of signs of their non-viability, an intestinal anastomosis is performed. Otherwise, a pathologically altered portion of the small bowel is resected.

During adhesiolysis, a surgeon may inadvertently damage the wall of the intestine, especially the dilated proximal portion. In this case, superficial slit-like defects of the serous layer should not be sutured, since after emptying the intestines their edges, as a rule, are converged by themselves. If not only the serous but also the muscle layer is damaged, seromuscular sutures should be applied with absorbable suture material on an atraumatic needle 4/0 or 5/0. If the intestinal lumen is accidentally opened, the perforated area is immediately plugged to prevent the release of contents. Strict adherence to the rules of aseptic technique is extremely important since the microflora located in the proximal dilated loop is always highly virulent. Therefore, in the case of abdominal contamination, there is a high risk of infectious postoperative complications. Before suturing, the damaged portion of the bowel should be separated from the surrounding adhesions and isolated from the abdominal cavity with gauze pads. Then, intestinal clamps are applied above and below the wound and the gauze pads are removed, the remnants of the intestinal contents are aspirated, and the site of perforation and adjacent tissues are treated with an antiseptic solution. The wound is sutured in the transverse direction with a double-row interrupted suture by using an absorbable suture material on an atraumatic needle 4/0–5/0.

After eliminating the obstruction, it is necessary to assess the viability of the portion of the small bowel involved in the pathological process. Absolute signs of its necrosis are a change in color to dark purple or black, absence of tone, peristalsis, pulsation of the mesenteric vessels and arteries of the intestinal wall, and specific putrefactive odor.

In doubtful cases, the altered bowel loop is immersed in the abdominal cavity and after 15–20 min its viability is checked. During this time, a surgeon may perform hemostasis, nasointestinal intubation, and aspirate intestinal contents. A more aggressive way is to warm a doubtful area with gauze pads moistened with hot saline. If these measures are not effective, the bowel is recognized as non-viable, which serves as an indication for its resection.

5. Resection of the gangrenous small bowel

Resection of the necrotic small intestine should be performed within healthy tissues to be sure that circulatory disturbances at the point of a cut are minimal. Considering more pronounced microcirculatory changes in the proximal loop, the cut should be 30–40 cm above and 15–20 cm below the site of visible necrosis. From a practical point of view, it should be noted that, due to the significant extensibility of the small bowel, it is impossible to determine the indicated length. Therefore, it is necessary to visually assess the condition of the mucous layer of the remaining bowel loops (color, bleeding, etc.). After resection, a side to side bowel anastomosis is the most appropriate. A two-row interrupted suture is applied with absorbable suture material on an atraumatic needle 4/0 or 5/0.

6. Nasointestinal intubation

The main indications for nasointestinal intubation in acute adhesive bowel obstruction are the dilation of the small bowel lumen for more than 5 cm and the need for its resection. An anesthetist in the operating room usually helps in installing the nasointestinal tube through the nose into the stomach. After this, the surgeon fixes the pylorus with the left hand and moves the tube tip through the stomach into the duodenal bulb with the right hand. Next, the tube is advanced through the duodenum by pushing its portion in the stomach. If the anatomy of the duodenum is normal, this maneuver may be done quite simply and quickly. However, if the duodenum is significantly deformed, the tube tip is slowly moved from the bulb into the vertical part of the duodenum. Then, the tube is advanced to the lower horizontal part of the duodenum with the right hand placed under the mesentery of the transverse colon. As a rule, from there the tube is easily moved beyond the Treitz ligament into the jejunum. This may not work out due to the deformation of the duodenojejunal transition, which should be eliminated. Forced tube advancement is unacceptable due to the danger of intestinal wall perforation.

When the nasointestinal tube tip passed the Treitz ligament, the tube is advanced through the small intestine, which is the easiest step of intubation. The operating surgeon moves the tube through the proximal part of the bowel, while the assistant straightens the bowel loops and directs the tube tip towards the ileocecal transition. At this step, it is necessary to avoid the formation of excessive tube loops in the stomach, which occur in the absence of synchronous actions of the surgeon and the anesthetist advancing the tube into the stomach. The tube tip should not be inserted into the cecum. The destruction of the ileocecal flap may cause colonic contents reflux and colonization of the small intestine by fecal microflora.

If the small intestine was resected, the tube tip is installed 30–50 cm distal to the intestinal anastomosis.

Intestinal aspiration is performed after intubation is completed. Next, it is necessary to verify the correct location of the nasointestinal tube, since the presence of loops, flexures, and deformations makes decompression ineffective. It is very important to determine the location of the last lateral perforation of the tube, which should be in the middle part of the stomach. Its displacement into the esophagus is strictly unacceptable, because it may lead to aspiration of the gastric contents into the respiratory tract in the postoperative period. A less dangerous mistake is to leave the last lateral perforation in the duodenum. In this case, patients may experience vomiting, as the cavity of the stomach is undrained. The tube may be marked with a narrow strip of adhesive tape near the last lateral perforation to facilitate its search.

At the end of the surgery, a surgeon should check hemostasis and remove the fluid from the abdominal cavity. The drainage tube is installed through a contraperture and placed in the pelvic cavity. The anterior abdominal wall layers are sutured with absorbable suture material.

I do not doubt that each experienced surgeon may offer personal original techniques that he or she uses during surgery for acute adhesive small bowel obstruction. Nevertheless, I would like to hope that the small nuances of the surgical technique described in this modest essay may help to avoid big problems during such surgical interventions.

Author details

Dmitry Garbuzenko
Department of Faculty Surgery, South Ural State Medical University, Chelyabinsk, Russia

*Address all correspondence to: garb@inbox.ru

References

[1] Garbuzenko DV. Selected Lectures in Emergency Abdominal Surgery. Saarbrücken, Germany: LAP LAMBERT Academic Publishing GmbH & Co.; 2012

[2] Ten Broek RPG, Krielen P, Di Saverio S, et al. Bologna guidelines for diagnosis and management of adhesive small bowel obstruction (ASBO): 2017 update of the evidence-based guidelines from the world society of emergency surgery ASBO working group. World Journal of Emergency Surgery. 2018;**13**:24

[3] Stich R, Makkas M. Fehler und Gefahren bei Chirurgischen Operationen. Mit 146 zum Teil Farbigen Abbildungen im Text und 2 Tafeln. Jena, Deutsch: Verlag: G. Fischer; 1923

Chapter 2

Adhesive Small Bowel Obstruction in the Minimally Invasive Era

Pepijn Krielen, Martijn W. J. Stommel,
Richard P. G. ten Broek and Harry van Goor

Abstract

Roughly 60% of all cases of small bowel obstruction are caused by adhesions. Adhesions are a form of internal scar tissue, which develop in over 45–93% of patients who undergo abdominal surgery. With this relatively high incidence, the population at risk for adhesive small bowel obstruction (ASBO) is enormous. Minimally invasive surgery reduces surgical wound surface and thus holds promise to reduce adhesion formation. The use of minimally invasive techniques results in a 50% reduction of adhesion formation as compared to open surgery. However, since ASBO can be caused by just a single adhesive band, it is uncertain whether a reduction in adhesion formation will also lead to a proportional decrease in the incidence of ASBO. Minimally invasive surgery might also improve operative treatment of ASBO, accelerating gastro-intestinal recovery time and lowering the risk of recurrent ASBO associated with adhesion reformation. We will discuss recent evidence on the impact of minimally invasive surgery on the incidence of ASBO and the role of minimally invasive surgery to resolve ASBO. Finally, we will debate additional measures, such as the use of adhesion barriers, to prevent adhesion formation and adhesion-related morbidity in the minimally invasive era.

Keywords: adhesions, adhesive small bowel obstruction, minimally invasive surgery, laparoscopy, adhesion barrier, adhesion reduction strategies

1. Introduction

As many as 60% of all episodes of small bowel obstruction (SBO) are caused by adhesions [1]. Adhesions are attachments of abdominal structures by internal scar tissue that are the result of healing of the peritoneum after it has been damaged, in most cases by surgery [2]. Adhesions can be filmy or dense and be present as an isolated band or as a 'curtain' or tangle with difficulty recognizing visceral structures. The degree of density and vascularization is traditionally classified using the Zühlke classification (**Table 1**) [3]. A more comprehensive and clinically relevant classification including projected locations of adhesions is the Peritoneal Adhesion Index (PAI) (**Figure 1**) [4, 5].

Adhesions develop in 89–93% of patients undergoing open abdominal or pelvic surgery [6, 7]. Incidence rates of adhesion formation are lower after minimally invasive surgery, 45–62% [7, 8]. Adhesions can also develop after other causes of peritoneal trauma, such as inflammatory conditions or radiotherapy [2].

Grade	Description
0	No adhesions or insignificant adhesions
I	Adhesions that are filmy and easy to separate by blunt dissection
II	Adhesions with beginning vascularization that can be dissected blunt but some sharp dissection is necessary
III	Adhesions with clear vascularization that can only be dissected using sharp dissection
IV	Adhesions which strongly attached organs, dissection is only possible by sharp dissection, damage of organs is hardly preventable

Adapted from Ref. [3].

Table 1.
Zühlke classification.

PERITONEAL ADHESION INDEX:

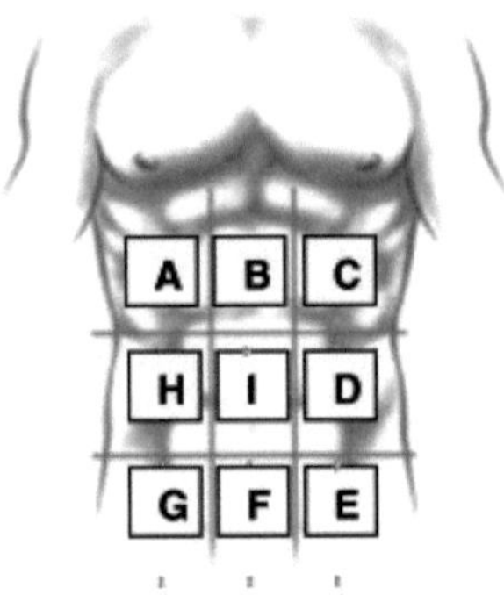

Regions:	Adhesion grade:
A Right upper	____
B Epigastrium	____
C Left upper	____
D Left flank	____
E Left lower	____
F Pelvis	____
G Right lower	____
H Right flank	____
I Central	____
L Bowel to bowel	____

Adhesion grade score:

0 No adhesions

1 Filmy adhesions, blunt dissection

2 Strong adhesions, sharp dissection

3 Very strong vascularized adhesions, sharp dissection, damage hardly preventable

PAI ☐

Figure 1.
Peritoneal adhesion index.

The occurrence of adhesions does not only cause a lifelong risk of adhesive small bowel obstruction (ASBO). Other clinical consequences of adhesions are difficulties during reoperation, female infertility, and chronic visceral pain; making it the most common cause of long-term complications in peritoneal surgery [1]. The incidence of ASBO is 2–3% in the first years after surgery in all patients who undergo abdominal or pelvic surgery [1]. The risk of ASBO depends on the anatomical location of surgery and the extent of surgery and peritoneal injury [1–10]. ASBO risk varies from 0.5% in abdominal wall surgery, 1.2% after upper gastrointestinal tract surgery to 3.2% in lower gastro-intestinal tract surgery and 4.2% in pediatric surgery [1].

Given the high incidence of adhesions and adhesion-related complications, one would assume that every surgeon is aware of the risks of adhesions. However, awareness on the full size of the problem only arose in response to the publication of the Surgical and Clinical Adhesion Research (SCAR) study two decades ago. The SCAR large population based study demonstrated that one of three patients undergoing abdominal surgery is readmitted for a cause possibly related to adhesions [11]. Subsequently adhesion-related complications gained increasing awareness of clinicians, hospitals and vendors, and adhesion reduction strategies were introduced. Laparoscopic surgeons hypothesized that minimally invasive surgical techniques would reduce peritoneal injury and thereby could solve the problem of adhesion formation. Other strategies to reduce adhesion formation were the development of adhesion barriers, the banishment of powdered gloves, and the introduction of new sealing devices [12].

Over the past decades, minimally invasive surgery has become the standard approach in many surgical disciplines. The rapid introduction of minimally invasive surgery was largely fueled by short-term benefits such as quicker recovery, reduced pain, and better cosmetic outcome [13]. Furthermore, surgeons strongly believed in the effectiveness of minimally invasive surgical techniques to reduce adhesion formation and subsequent morbidity [14]. For this reasons adhesion barriers are only seldomly used in minimally invasive surgery [15], and are believed to be needed only in open surgery. Despite good evidence of effective reduction of adhesion formation and subsequent adhesion-related morbidity, the use of adhesion barriers in open surgery is also limited [16]. Reasons for not using adhesion barriers are the lack of trust in adhesion reduction, the expected limited impact on adhesion-related complications, and the costs of the barriers [15]. The limited use of adhesion barriers has slowed down the research and development of adhesion-prevention strategies in the past decade.

Studies on adhesion formation in minimally invasive surgery report a reduction of approximately 50% in the extent of postoperative adhesions compared with open surgery [7]. Unfortunately, trials comparing open and minimally invasive surgery have not been designed and powered to compare long-term adhesion-related outcomes [17]. Therefore, the effect of the broad implementation of minimally invasive surgery on clinically relevant outcome parameters such as ASBO and readmissions is unknown [17]. A reduction in adhesion formation, does not necessarily correlate with a proportionate reduction in the risk of ASBO; a single adhesive band may cause a life-threatening bowel obstruction, whereas extensive dense abdominal adhesions may be asymptomatic [18]. Nevertheless, potential benefits of minimally invasive surgery in preventing adhesion-related morbidity seem compelling.

Minimally invasive surgery may also play a role in the treatment of ASBO. Approximately 25% of patients with ASBO require surgery to resolve the bowel obstruction [1], and recurrence rates are high [19]. The minimally invasive approach is hypothesized to accelerate recovery, and might also reduce risk of regrowth of adhesions and subsequent recurrence of ASBO. A caveat is the small working space and vulnerability of the bowel caused by the distention of the obstructed bowel that could result in iatrogenic injuries. In this chapter, we discuss recent evidence on the effects of the introduction of minimally invasive surgery on the burden of adhesions and ASBO. We further discuss the role of minimally invasive surgery in the treatment of patients with ASBO. We end with a contemplation on the awareness of adhesion-related complications and the value of adhesion barriers in minimally invasive surgery.

2. The problem of adhesive small bowel obstruction

The vast majority of adhesions develop after abdominal or pelvic surgery, although adhesions can also form after abdominal and pelvic radiation and peritoneal inflammation [2]. Adhesions are associated with a lifelong risk of ASBO. Incidence and morbidity of ASBO might be somewhat difficult to estimate and compare between studies based on different definitions for ASBO. Most accepted definition of ASBO is an episode of SBO with the presence of adhesions confirmed during reoperation. However, operative confirmation of adhesions is often not possible because many ASBO episodes are managed non-operatively. Therefore a second definition of ASBO is commonly applied: an episode of SBO interpreted as matching ASBO on radiological imaging after excluding other potential causes of bowel obstruction e.g. hernia, tumor, bezoar.

In a systematic review, the incidence of SBO by any cause after surgery is estimated 9% [1]. In 42 etiological studies on SBO, adhesions accounted for 56% of all SBO episodes, either by operative confirmation or by excluding all other potential causes of SBO [1]. The incidence of postoperative ASBO confirmed by surgery is estimated at 2.4%. Depending on the type of initial surgical procedure, the incidence varied between 0.5 and 4.2% [1]. As mentioned, this estimate is conservative because most episodes of ASBO are managed non-operative.

Another way to estimate the burden of ASBO is based on population studies. In the SCAR study more than one in three patients were readmitted for a cause possibly related to adhesions, and more than 1 in 20 patients (6%) who underwent open abdominal or pelvic surgery were readmitted for a directly adhesion-related cause [11]. The most common diagnosis for a directly adhesion-related readmission was ASBO [11]. More recent population studies in the UK and USA show that ASBO remains a major contributor to the morbidity, mortality and costs related to emergency abdominal surgery. In the UK in 2016, 51% of all emergency laparotomies were for ASBO [20]. Similar results were found in the USA between 2008 and 2011, where SBO needing adhesiolysis belonged to the top 5 of emergency surgical procedures [21]. Given these numbers and the number of patients undergoing abdominal or pelvic surgery, the impact of ASBO on a population level is high.

ASBO causes significant morbidity and a hospital admission for SBO is associated with 2.5% mortality [1]. Initial non-operative management of ASBO includes gastric decompression, fluid resuscitation and nil per os, which is successful in 70–90% [1–23]. In a sizable number of cases ASBO will result in emergency or delayed, after failed initial conservative management, abdominal surgery. Open or minimally invasive adhesiolysis to resolve the obstruction is associated with a incidence of 6–20% enterotomies [24, 25]. In general, complex adhesiolysis is associated with bleeding, sepsis, wound infections and increased mortality, even in the absence of bowel injury [26]. Mean length of hospital stay for ASBO ranges from 4 to 13 days and generally depends the type of treatment and the treatment complications [1].

Both operative and conservative management of ASBO are associated with a risk of recurrent ASBO. Operative management includes repeated peritoneal injury with risk of adhesion reformation and re-ASBO. Non-operative management of ASBO does not dissolve abdominal adhesions and harbors the risk of a new episode of ASBO. In a recent study of patients presenting with a first episode of ASBO, operative management was associated with a lower risk of recurrence compared with non-operative management (13% vs. 21%) after a median follow-up of 3.6 years [19]. The study also showed an increased risk of ASBO with every previous episode of ASBO in accordance to findings done 25 years ago [27]. Also the time between episodes of ASBO decreases with an increase in number of episodes [19]. Despite the higher recurrence rate after conservative treatment, current guidelines still recommend a trial of non-operative management of ASBO in order to avoid the risk of complications associated with surgical intervention [28].

Effort is made to predict the severity of ASBO using peri-operative scores [29, 30]. However, the scores are not widely adopted for clinical use. The American Association for the Surgery of Trauma (AAST) developed a score based on clinical, imaging, operative and pathologic criteria to grade disease severity of ASBO [31, 32]. The AAST grade uses clinical criteria (flatus, bowel sounds abdominal distention), pathologic criteria (bowel perforation), imaging criteria on CT (intestinal distention, transition point, contrast flow) and operative criteria (intestinal distention, impeding bowel compromise, peritonitis) to define the grade of ASBO on a scale from 1 to 4. A higher AAST score for emergency ASBO is associated with an increase in length of hospital stay, pneumonia, and more severe complications [33]. Recently the Clinical Adhesion Score (CLAS) was developed, measuring the full spectrum of the long-term burden of adhesion formation in post-operative patients. CLAS calculates the overall morbidity based on four domains: ASBO, difficulties during reoperation, female infertility or subfertility, and chronic abdominal pain (data not yet published). Evaluation of current and new adhesion prevention strategies regarding long-term clinical efficacy e.g. ASBO could benefit from using CLAS.

The economic burden of ASBO is high. Operative management is the single most important determinant of costs. However, based on fewer recurrences of ASBO after surgical treatment, surgery may save costs at the long term [34]. Several studies have been reported regarding the treatment costs of ASBO. Most have important limitations reporting part of the costs or costs based on reimbursement prices rather than true healthcare costs [35–37]. We modeled in a recent study, costs for ASBO in the Netherlands using a micro-costing method including costs of length of stay, ICU days, operative time, medication, parenteral feeding, imaging studies and laboratory studies [38]. This modeling revealed total healthcare costs of patients operated for ASBO of €16305 (SD €2513) with a mean hospital stay of 16.0 ± 11 days. For non-operatively treated patients costs would be €2277 (SD €265) with a mean hospital stay of 4.0 ± 2.0 days. The majority of the costs were due to ward stay, operative time, ICU stay and (parental) feeding. All surgical procedures for ASBO in this study consisted of open adhesiolysis. Costs estimated in this study were higher compared to previous estimates of treatment costs for ASBO with comparable lengths of stay and, as a result of its design better reflecting reality [35–37]. In the study we adhered to international guidelines for the diagnosis and treatment of ASBO increasing generalizability of outcomes for developed countries.

Nevertheless costs may vary among countries due to differences in admission and discharge policies, and prices of diagnostics, materials, medication and feeding.

3. Impact of minimally invasive surgery on morbidity of ASBO

It has been suggested from a few studies that the decreased adhesion formation after minimally invasive surgery associates with a lower incidence of ASBO. This decrease seems limited compared to open surgery as concluded from one systematic review and one trial reported by our group [1–17]. Differences in definitions of ASBO used, types of procedures, outcome parameters and length of follow-up in the studies, preclude a firm conclusion on the beneficial effect of minimally invasive surgery on development of ASBO.

To estimate the impact of minimally invasive surgery at a population level on adhesion-related complications, ASBO in particular, our group recently reported the results of the SCAR update study [39]. Over 72,000 patients, who were operated between June 2009 and June 2011, were followed for a minimum of 5 years. Readmissions were classified, according to the initial SCAR study (1999), as directly-related to adhesions e.g. adhesive small bowel obstruction, possibly related to adhesions, e.g. any small bowel obstruction and reoperations potentially complicated by adhesions e.g. right hemicolectomy years after an appendectomy. Approximately 30% of all index procedures were minimally invasive. Patients who underwent minimally invasive surgery were readmitted less frequently for directly related causes compared with patients after open surgery (1.7% vs. 4.3%). Possibly related readmissions and reoperations potentially complicated by adhesions were also less frequent (16.0% vs. 18.2% and 8.6% vs. 15.0%). Multivariate analysis revealed a 32% reduction in directly adhesion-related readmissions associated with minimally invasive surgery. Readmission rates were similar when comparing patients with open surgery in the SCAR and those in the SCAR update study. The overall small differences found in readmission rates could be explained by the difference in follow-up, 10 years in the SCAR study and 5 years in the SCAR update study. Despite the finding of a small reduction in readmission rates after initial minimally invasive surgery, the overall burden of adhesion-related readmissions on a population level remains high.

To further elaborate differences in adhesion-related readmissions between minimally invasive and open surgery, we analyzed patients with colorectal procedures (data not yet published). This type of surgery is known for its adhesion formation propensity and associated morbidity. Over 15,000 patients underwent colorectal surgery of whom almost one-third with a minimally invasive approach. For open colorectal surgery readmission rates were comparable between the SCAR study and the SCAR update study. Minimally invasive colonic and/or rectal surgery reduced the total number of directly adhesion-related readmissions. However in patients who underwent a (sub)total colectomy readmission rates were over 15% irrespective of an open or minimally invasive approach. Minimally invasive surgery did not reduce adhesion-related complications in rectal procedures. We concluded that an extended colectomy and rectal resection do not benefit from minimally invasive surgery regarding adhesion-related complications. We hypothesized that the large extent of the dissection and injury to the visceral and lateral parietal peritoneum needed in both surgical techniques abolishes the preventive effect of the minimally invasive technique on adhesion formation to the ventral peritoneum, where the injury is relatively limited for both approaches.

The SCAR update study has demonstrated that minimally invasive surgery is associated with less adhesion-related readmissions. Hence, the overall burden of adhesion-related readmissions on a population level remains high. Adhesion formation therefore continues to be a challenge in abdominal surgery, also in the minimally invasive era. Minimally invasive procedures were only performed in approximately one-third of procedures in 2009–2011, whereas currently in the Netherlands about 75% of colonic resections are performed minimally invasive (by laparoscopy or robot) [40]. On a population base a further decline in adhesion-related complications can be expected with an increase of minimally invasive abdominal operations. However, we like to warn against unbridled optimism regarding the overall impact of minimally invasive surgery on the burden of adhesions because open surgery is still being preferred when a complicated condition is expected in the abdominal cavity e.g. after multiple previous procedures, with large inflammatory mass or locally advanced cancer [41]. Many of these conditions are complex specifically due to presence of adhesions at baseline surgery and the need to perform adhesiolysis before entering the operative area. It is known that the propensity to reform adhesions after adhesiolysis is higher than de novo adhesion formation.

4. Management of adhesive small bowel obstruction

Adequate management of ASBO depends on an initially correct diagnosis. Although ASBO is a common diagnosis with clear signs and symptoms, misdiagnosis and delayed diagnosis are a substantial clinical problem. Up to 50% of older patients are initially not adequately diagnosed [42]. Failure to diagnose represents 70% of malpractice claims in ASBO [43, 44]. In this regard it is important to note that patients with ASBO can initially present themselves to a variety of physicians, including general practitioners, surgeons, internal medicine physicians, geriatricians and gastroenterologists. To improve diagnosis of ASBO, multiple specialists need to be involved in practice guidelines and protocols.

Based on expert opinion the diagnosing of ASBO includes a medical history with an assessment of potential causes of SBO, e.g. previous abdominal surgery, inflammatory bowel disease, important symptoms such as vomiting, absence of stools or flatus, intermittent colicky abdominal pain and abdominal distention. Common pitfalls in diagnosing ASBO are the less prominent pain present in the elderly [42], reporting of watery diarrhea by patients with an incomplete obstruction and normal stool passage in the first days after onset due to stool still present in the colon.

The recent update of the international guidelines for diagnosis and management of ASBO gives the current best available evidence for management of ASBO once the diagnosis of bowel obstruction has been established [28]. The first priority in management is to establish the cause of obstruction and to determine if urgent surgical treatment is required. ASBO is the single most common cause for SBO, the differential diagnosis includes strangulated abdominal wall or groin hernia, tumor, paralysis, constipation or bezoars. Laboratory tests should include blood count, CRP, electrolytes, creatinine and lactate. Imaging studies can include water-soluble contrast studies or computer tomography (CT) scans. CT scan is the preferred imaging technique for the diagnosis of ASBO, it can accurately rule out other causes of obstruction and identify patients who might require emergency surgery [28]. Water-soluble contrast enhances the diagnostic accuracy of CT scans. Signs that might suspect ASBO on imaging studies are an abrupt change in bowel diameter and the exclusion of other causes of SBO. The value of plain X-rays is limited [28].

Urgent surgery is required in case of signs of ischemia, perforation or strangulation of the bowel, generalized peritonitis and/or hemodynamic instability. No single test is highly sensitive for ischemia and strangulation. Sensitivity of physical examination for the detection of strangulation is only 48% in experienced hands [45]. Laboratory tests indicating peritonitis or ischemia are a CRP above 75 and a white blood cell count above 10.000/mm^3 [45–47]. Again, a CT scan is most accurate in assessing strangulation and perforation and the need for emergency surgery [28]. CT abnormalities indicating strangulation or perforation are free intraperitoneal air or fluid, closed loop obstruction, mesenteric edema or engorgement, mesenteric swirling, pneumatosis intestinalis, decreased or lack of bowel enhancement or thickened bowel wall [48–50].

If bowel obstruction is caused by adhesions, and signs of peritonitis, ischemia, and strangulation are absent, initial conservative treatment is reportedly safe. Conservative treatment is successful in 70–90% of all episodes of ASBO [1–23]. Conservative treatment of ASBO consists of nil per os and decompression of the gastro-intestinal tract using a naso-gastric tube. Further management includes fluid resuscitation, correction of electrolyte disturbances, nutritional support and prevention of aspiration. Optimal duration of a conservative trial is debated; prolonged management for more than 72 h has been associated with adverse outcomes and increased mortality [20, 51–54]. Water-soluble contrast studies seem useful in the follow-up of conservative management of ASBO. If contrast has not reached to colon 24–48 h following administration, continuation of conservative management is likely to fail and surgical management should be considered [28].

An algorithm for the diagnosis and treatment of ASBO is presented in **Figure 2** [28].

4.1 Role of minimally invasive surgery in the management of ASBO

Operative treatment of ASBO historically comprises an explorative laparotomy with adhesiolysis. The increased use of minimally invasive surgery has raised the question whether minimally invasive surgery is feasible and effective for the treatment of ASBO. Benefits of minimally invasive adhesiolysis are reduction of peritoneal injury possibly resulting in less adhesion reformation, a quick recovery and minimal post-operative pain. Twenty-five years ago the first cases of minimally invasive surgery for treatment of ASBO have been described [55]. Thereafter a few series were reported but adequate comparative trials are scarce [56–60]. Minimally invasive surgery for ASBO is challenging because there is little laparoscopic working space due to the distended bowel. Also visibility can be hampered by multiple adhesions. There are concerns that minimally invasive surgery increases the risk of iatrogenic bowel perforations [57]. Suitability of minimally invasive surgery for ASBO further depends on patient characteristics. In case of hemodynamic instability open surgery is required because patients cannot tolerate the pneumoperitoneum.

One randomized trial comparing minimally invasive and open surgery for ASBO has been performed [56]. Only patients with a high suspicion of a single adhesive band causing the obstruction were included. Patients with confirmed or suspected peritoneal carcinosis, known multiple adhesions, previous open surgery for endometriosis, aorta, iliac vessels or Crohn's disease, previous generalized peritonitis, abdominal malignancy, previous abdominal radiotherapy or recent operations within 30 days were all excluded. Patients started with conservative management of ASBO. If the obstruction did not resolve patients were randomized between open and laparoscopic adhesiolysis. The trial was open label, therefore patients and care providers were not blinded. During 5 years 566 patients were included in the study, 104 patients underwent surgery, 51 were randomly assigned to the open surgery

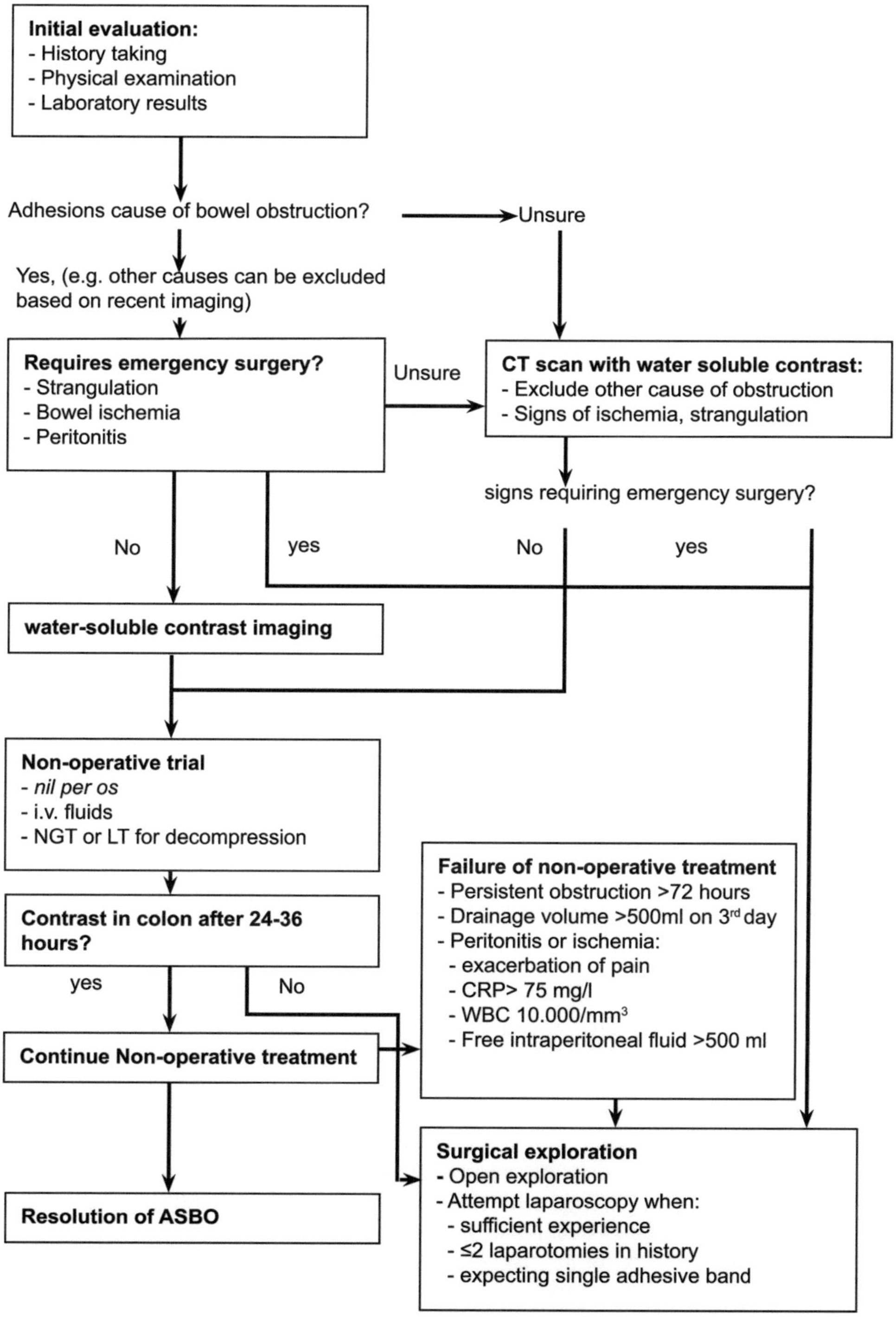

Figure 2.
Algorithm for the diagnosis and treatment of ASBO.

group, and 53 to the laparoscopic surgery group. Patients in the laparoscopic group had a shorter length of stay (4.2 days) compared with the open group (5.5 days). Mortality and postoperative complications did not differ between the groups.

The few matched cohort studies comparing minimally invasive and open surgery for ASBO reported comparable results to those of the trial mentioned above

[59, 60]. There seems a trend towards a faster recovery in selected patients. Studies showed no major differences in complications or mortality. A few studies specifically addressed the potential drawbacks of the minimally invasive approach and suggested an increased risk of bowel injury [59]. Notably, the non-matched cohorts frequently claim large beneficial effects of the laparoscopic approach [40–58]. However, these studies have a high risk of various types of selection bias, mainly excluding patients who are more sick or are suspected of multiple adhesions.

It seems that minimally invasive adhesiolysis holds promise for patients with signs of a single adhesive band and an uncomplicated disease course. Further studies are needed to identify patients who can benefit from minimally invasive adhesiolysis and patients who can be harmed by minimally invasive treatment for ASBO.

5. Future perspectives

5.1 Awareness of adhesions formation by minimally invasive surgery

Morbidity of adhesion formation in minimally invasive surgery is often underestimated. Less than 25% of surgeons and 5–83% of gynecologists routinely inform their patients about adhesions and the life term risk of adhesion-related complications [14–62]. However, recent evidence shows that adhesion-related morbidity remains high in the minimally invasive era [39]. Not informing patients about the risk of adhesions might therefore be considered negligent. Increased awareness of adhesions might create an urge for the development and refinement of adhesion prevention strategies.

Awareness of adhesions may improve by growing awareness for intra-operative complications in general. Impact of adhesions on the operative course of reoperations for ASBO or other indications is often underreported. In a prospective comparison of operative notes and observation by an independent researcher, one in seven iatrogenic bowel injuries was not reported in operative notes, and almost one in three minor injuries [63]. In recent years, there is increasing scientific interest in the consequences of intra-operative events. IAEs are associated with 40% more hospital admissions, a twofold higher readmission rate, and with worse post-operative outcome [64–70]. Recently the Classification of Intraoperative Complications (CLASSIC) has been developed as a new tool for systematic classification for intra-operative complications (iAEs) [71]. CLASSIC defines iAEs as any deviation from the ideal intraoperative course, including technical failures, surgical and anesthesiological difficulties. The score has been update to five grades of severity (https://clinicaltrials.gov/ct2/show/NCT03009929). Lysis of adhesions at reoperations is associated with post-operative increase of sepsis, intra-abdominal complications, wound infections, longer hospital stay, and higher hospital costs [26–72]. As such, adhesiolysis qualifies as an iAE if adhesiolysis is not the intended surgical procedure. We currently investigate the contribution of adhesiolysis and associated intra-operative complications e.g. bleeding, inadvertent enterotomy to the CLASSIC.

Recent published guidelines may also increase awareness of adhesions and treatment of ASBO [28]. An old saying on ASBO is 'you must not let the sun rise on ASBO', all patients presenting with ASBO were operated if conservative management failed to resolve the bowel obstruction within 24 h. Recent insights report that a conservative trial can safely be prolonged to 72 h [51, 52]. The current guideline states that conservative treatment should be instigated in all patients without signs of ischemia, perforation or strangulation of the bowel, generalized peritonitis and/or hemodynamic instability [28]. Contradictory, some studies report lower recurrence rates of ASBO after surgical management of ASBO [19–27]. A further disadvantage of prolonged conservative management is the further clinical deterioration of highly comorbid patients who receive starvation treatment for a few days [73]. Minimally invasive surgery could change the paradigm again towards earlier surgical intervention because of faster recovery, reduced length of hospital stay and the mentioned lower recurrence rates of ASBO.

5.2 Adhesion reduction strategies

Considering the high impact of adhesion-related complications on a population level that is not substantially decreased by minimally invasive surgery, there is a pressing need to develop new adhesion reduction strategies.

Until now the most promising approach for reduction of adhesion formation is routinely applying an adhesion barrier. Adhesion barriers are bioresorbable liquids, gels or films that keep injured peritoneal wound surfaces separated. During separation the peritoneal wound can heal with restoration of peritoneal tissue morphology and function without 'scarring' (adhesions). A large systematic review and meta-analysis in 2014 of 28 trials (n = 5191) showed benefits of several adhesion barriers in predominantly open abdominal surgery [16]. However, adhesion barriers are seldomly applied in abdominal or pelvic surgery [14]. Only 1 in 7 surgeons ever uses adhesion barriers [14]. Reluctance of surgeons to use adhesions barriers seems caused by doubts about cost-effectiveness and the need and possibility of adhesion prevention in minimally invasive surgery.

Cost-effectiveness of adhesion prevention in minimally invasive surgery is an important perquisite for implementation in every day practice. We performed a modeling study on cost-effectiveness of adhesion barriers in minimally invasive procedures with a high risk of adhesion formation [74]. Two strategies were compared: current clinical practice (colorectal surgery without the use of an adhesion barrier) and colorectal surgery with the use of an adhesion barrier (hyaluronate carboxymethylcellulose). Whilst hyaluronate carboxymethylcellulose as such is not applicable in minimally invasive surgery and a gel form has not properly been studied in minimally invasive surgery, probabilities were extrapolated from data of open colorectal surgery. Probability estimates were derived from literature. Costs of treatment of ASBO were derived from our previous report [38]. Cost of hyaluronate carboxymethylcellulose was estimated on $630, based on the mean number of films used in studies on hyaluronate carboxymethylcellulose [12–75]. We concluded that using an adhesion barrier was more effective than not using a barrier in minimally invasive surgery, but it was more expensive. However, mean expected direct healthcare costs in the 4 years following index surgery increased with only $163 per patient. Cost estimates in this modeling study only included direct health care costs. Societal costs (e.g. absence from work) were not modeled in this study. Therefore an increase of $163 in direct health care may be neglectable considering potential gain in societal costs. Further research is needed on long term savings regarding socio-economic costs with adhesion barriers also including the new SCAR update data of minimally invasive surgery.

An important limitation of most barriers is the inability to properly use these in minimally invasive surgery. Most barriers were developed more than two to three decades ago and were films intended for use in open surgery. This limitation and the disregard needing barriers in minimally invasive surgery have impeded implementation and continued research and development of barriers suitable for minimally invasive surgery (and open surgery). Recently some new barriers have been developed suitable for minimally invasive surgery. Studies on these new barriers are performed mostly in gynecologic populations, and show effectiveness reducing adhesions [76, 77]. The important next step in adhesion prevention is the development of a new generation of barriers suitable for minimally invasive use in general surgery [78, 79]. Using increased knowledge of the pathophysiology of adhesions, new barriers consist of bioactive and targeted technology e.g. modulation of inflammation [2]. Pilpel and colleagues developed a liquid solution modulating the fibrin matrix which is generated by the hemostatic system after peritoneal injury [80]. This novel therapy is currently tested in animal models. Roberston and colleagues are testing a drug (L-Alanyl-L-Glutamine) to regulate the formation of adhesions due to hypoxia and oxidative stress caused by surgical injury of the vascular supply to the tissue caused by surgical intervention [81]. The first results of this drug in a double-blinded placebo controlled study show that L-Alanyl-L-Glutamine is safe to use and is effective at reducing adhesion formation after laparoscopic myomectomies [82]. Definitive results from this study are expected in due time. When proven safe, effective and affordable in patients, these new bioactive and targeted technology agents should be administered during index minimally invasive surgery to break the sequence of intra- and postoperative adhesion-(re) formation related complications.

6. Conclusions

Adhesion-related morbidity remains a clinically relevant problem in the minimally invasive era. Minimally invasive surgery is associated with only a modest reduction in adhesion-related readmissions and incidence of ASBO. The growing body of scientific evidence provides the clinician with a firm guideline for the diagnosis and treatment of ASBO. Minimally invasive surgery in the management of ASBO appears to be safe and effective alternative to open adhesiolysis, however in a very selected patient group. To allow as many patients as possible to benefit from a minimally invasive approach future research should focus on the selection criteria for minimally invasive surgery in ASBO. Adhesion-related morbidity is often underestimated and complications of adhesiolysis underreported. Raising awareness of adhesions therefore remains important. Using newly proposed scores for intraoperative complications, may increase awareness for the intra-operative events caused by adhesions. Adhesion barriers can safely reduce adhesion formation, are cost-effective in open colorectal surgery and effective with slightly higher costs in minimally invasive surgery. Future research should focus on new bioactive barriers that are easily applicable in minimally invasive abdominal surgery and safe to use. Preventing adhesions during first minimally invasive surgery is key to break the sequence of intra- and postoperative adhesion (re)formation related complications.

Conflict of interest

The authors declare no conflict of interest.

Author details

Pepijn Krielen*, Martijn W. J. Stommel, Richard P. G. ten Broek and Harry van Goor
Department of Surgery, Radboud University Medical Center, Nijmegen,
The Netherlands

*Address all correspondence to: pepijn.krielen@radboudumc.nl

References

[1] ten Broek RP et al. Burden of adhesions in abdominal and pelvic surgery: Systematic review and met-analysis. BMJ. 2013;**347**:f5588

[2] Stommel MW, Strik C, van Goor H. Response to pathological processes in the peritoneal cavity—Sepsis, tumours, adhesions, and ascites. Seminars in Pediatric Surgery. 2014;**23**(6):331-335

[3] Zuhlke HV et al. Pathophysiology and classification of adhesions. Langenbecks Archiv für Chirurgie. Supplement II, Verhandlungen der Deutschen Gesellschaft für Chirurgie. Deutsche Gesellschaft für Chirurgie. 1990:1009-1016. Available from: https://www.ncbi.nlm.nih.gov/pubmed/?term=1983476

[4] Coccolini F et al. Peritoneal adhesion index (PAI): Proposal of a score for the "ignored iceberg" of medicine and surgery. World Journal of Emergency Surgery. 2013;**8**(1):6

[5] Fugazzola P et al. Validation of peritoneal adhesion index as a standardized classification to universalize peritoneal adhesions definition. Journal of Peritoneum (and Other Serosal Surfaces). 2017;**2**:61-69

[6] Menzies D, Ellis H. Intestinal obstruction from adhesions—How big is the problem? Annals of the Royal College of Surgeons of England. 1990;**72**(1):60-63

[7] Stommel MWJ et al. Multicenter observational study of adhesion formation after open- and laparoscopic surgery for colorectal cancer. Annals of Surgery. 2018;**267**(4):743-748

[8] Polymeneas G et al. A comparative study of postoperative adhesion formation after laparoscopic vs open cholecystectomy. Surgical Endoscopy. 2001;**15**(1):41-43

[9] Parker MC et al. Colorectal surgery: The risk and burden of adhesion-related complications. Colorectal Disease. 2004;**6**(6):506-511

[10] Barmparas G et al. The incidence and risk factors of post-laparotomy adhesive small bowel obstruction. Journal of Gastrointestinal Surgery. 2010;**14**(10):1619-1628

[11] Ellis H et al. Adhesion-related hospital readmissions after abdominal and pelvic surgery: A retrospective cohort study. Lancet. 1999;**353**(9163):1476-1480

[12] Ten Broek RP et al. Different surgical techniques to reduce post-operative adhesion formation: A systematic review and meta-analysis. Human Reproduction Update. 2013;**19**(1):12-25

[13] Kuhry E et al. Long-term results of laparoscopic colorectal cancer resection. Cochrane Database of Systematic Reviews. 2008;**2**:CD003432

[14] van Steensel S et al. Adhesion awareness in 2016: An update of the national survey of surgeons. PLoS One. 2018;**13**(8):e0202418

[15] Schreinemacher MH et al. Adhesion awareness: A national survey of surgeons. World Journal of Surgery. 2010;**34**(12):2805-2812

[16] Ten Broek RPG et al. Benefits and harms of adhesion barriers for abdominal surgery: A systematic review and meta-analysis. Lancet. 2014;**383**(9911):48-59

[17] Yamada T et al. Meta-analysis of the risk of small bowel obstruction following open or laparoscopic colorectal surgery. The British Journal of Surgery. 2016;**103**(5):493-503

[18] Diamond MP et al. Adhesion prevention and reduction: Current status and future recommendations of a multinational interdisciplinary consensus conference. Surgical Innovation. 2010;**17**(3):183-188

[19] Behman R et al. Association of surgical intervention for adhesive small-bowel obstruction with the risk of recurrence. JAMA Surgery. 2019;**154**(5):413-420

[20] NELA Project Team. The Third Patient Report of the National Emergency Laparotomy Audit (NELA). London: The Royal College of Anaesthetists; 2017

[21] Scott JW et al. Use of national burden to define operative emergency general surgery. JAMA Surgery. 2016;**151**(6):e160480

[22] Fazel MZ, Jamieson RW, Watson CJ. Long-term follow-up of the use of the Jones' intestinal tube in adhesive small bowel obstruction. Annals of the Royal College of Surgeons of England. 2009;**91**(1):50-54

[23] Schraufnagel D, Rajaee S, Millham FH. How many sunsets? Timing of surgery in adhesive small bowel obstruction: A study of the nationwide inpatient sample. Journal of Trauma and Acute Care Surgery. 2013;**74**(1):181-187. discussion 187-9

[24] Wullstein C, Gross E. Laparoscopic compared with conventional treatment of acute adhesive small bowel obstruction. The British Journal of Surgery. 2003;**90**(9):1147-1151

[25] Fevang BT et al. Long-term prognosis after operation for adhesive small bowel obstruction. Annals of Surgery. 2004;**240**(2):193-201

[26] ten Broek RP et al. Adhesiolysis-related morbidity in abdominal surgery. Annals of Surgery. 2013;**258**(1):98-106

[27] Barkan H, Webster S, Ozeran S. Factors predicting the recurrence of adhesive small-bowel obstruction. American Journal of Surgery. 1995;**170**(4):361-365

[28] Ten Broek RPG et al. Bologna guidelines for diagnosis and management of adhesive small bowel obstruction (ASBO): 2017 update of the evidence-based guidelines from the world society of emergency surgery ASBO working group. World Journal of Emergency Surgery. 2018;**13**:24

[29] Zielinski MD et al. Small bowel obstruction—Who needs an operation? A multivariate prediction model. World Journal of Surgery. 2010;**34**(5):910-919

[30] Jancelewicz T et al. Predicting strangulated small bowel obstruction: An old problem revisited. Journal of Gastrointestinal Surgery. 2009;**13**(1):93-99

[31] Shafi S et al. Measuring anatomic severity of disease in emergency general surgery. Journal of Trauma and Acute Care Surgery. 2014;**76**(3):884-887

[32] Utter GH et al. ICD-9-CM and ICD-10-CM mapping of the AAST emergency general surgery disease severity grading systems: Conceptual approach, limitations, and recommendations for the future. Journal of Trauma and Acute Care Surgery. 2015;**78**(5):1059-1065

[33] Hernandez MC et al. Application of the AAST EGS grade for adhesive small bowel obstruction to a multi-national patient population. World Journal of Surgery. 2018;**42**(11):3581-3588

[34] Colonna AL et al. Nonoperative management of adhesive small bowel obstruction: What is the break point? American Journal of Surgery. 2016;**212**(6):1214-1221

[35] Shapter SL, Paul MJ, White SM. Incidence and estimated annual cost of emergency laparotomy in England: Is there a major funding shortfall? Anaesthesia. 2012;**67**(5):474-478

[36] ten Broek RP et al. Epidemiology and prevention of postsurgical adhesions revisited. Annals of Surgery. 2016;**263**(1):12-19

[37] Wilson MS. Practicalities and costs of adhesions. Colorectal Disease. 2007;**9**(Suppl 2):60-65

[38] Krielen P et al. In-hospital costs of an admission for adhesive small bowel obstruction. World Journal of Emergency Surgery. 2016;**11**:49

[39] Krielen P et al. Adhesion-related readmissions after open and laparoscopic surgery: A retrospective cohort study (SCAR update). Lancet. 2020;**395**(10217):33-41

[40] Behman R et al. Laparoscopic surgery for adhesive small bowel obstruction is associated with a higher risk of bowel injury: A population-based analysis of 8584 patients. Annals of Surgery. 2017;**266**(3):489-498

[41] Licciardello A et al. Preoperative risk factors for conversion from laparoscopic to open cholecystectomy. European Review for Medical and Pharmacological Sciences. 2014;**18** (2 Suppl):60-68

[42] Ozturk E et al. Small bowel obstruction in the elderly: A plea for comprehensive acute geriatric care. World Journal of Emergency Surgery. 2018;**13**:48

[43] Ellis H, Crowe A. Medico-legal consequences of post-operative intra-abdominal adhesions. International Journal of Surgery. 2009;**7**(3):187-191

[44] Choudhry AJ et al. Medical malpractice in the management of small bowel obstruction: A 33-year review of case law. Surgery. 2016;**160**(4):1017-1027

[45] Sarr MG, Bulkley GB, Zuidema GD. Preoperative recognition of intestinal strangulation obstruction. Prospective evaluation of diagnostic capability. American Journal of Surgery. 1983;**145**(1):176-182

[46] Krause WR, Webb TP. Geriatric small bowel obstruction: An analysis of treatment and outcomes compared with a younger cohort. American Journal of Surgery. 2015;**209**(2):347-351

[47] Shih SC et al. Adhesive small bowel obstruction: How long can patients tolerate conservative treatment? World Journal of Gastroenterology. 2003;**9**(3):603-605

[48] Zielinski MD et al. Prospective, observational validation of a multivariate small-bowel obstruction model to predict the need for operative intervention. Journal of the American College of Surgeons. 2011;**212**(6):1068-1076

[49] Millet I et al. Assessment of strangulation in adhesive small bowel obstruction on the basis of combined CT findings: Implications for clinical care. Radiology. 2017;**285**(3):798-808

[50] Millet I et al. Value of CT findings to predict surgical ischemia in small bowel obstruction: A systematic review and meta-analysis. European Radiology. 2015;**25**(6):1823-1835

[51] Sakakibara T et al. The indicator for surgery in adhesive small bowel obstruction patient managed with long tube. Hepato-Gastroenterology. 2007;**54**(75):787-790

[52] Keenan JE et al. Trials of nonoperative management exceeding 3 days are associated with increased morbidity in patients undergoing surgery for uncomplicated adhesive

small bowel obstruction. Journal of Trauma and Acute Care Surgery. 2014;**76**(6):1367-1372

[53] Fevang BT et al. Early operation or conservative management of patients with small bowel obstruction? The European Journal of Surgery. 2002;**168**(8-9):475-481

[54] Foster NM et al. Small bowel obstruction: A population-based appraisal. Journal of the American College of Surgeons. 2006;**203**(2):170-176

[55] Mouret P. L'adesiolisi coelioscopia. In: Testas P, Delaitre B, editors. Chirurgia digestiva per via coelioscopica. Edizioni Vigot, Friburgo; 1994. pp. 53-69

[56] Sallinen V et al. Laparoscopic versus open adhesiolysis for adhesive small bowel obstruction (LASSO): An international, multicentre, randomised, open-label trial. The Lancet Gastroenterology & Hepatology. 2019;**4**(4):278-286

[57] Di Saverio S et al. Laparoscopic adhesiolysis: Not for all patients, not for all surgeons, not in all centres. Updates in Surgery. 2018;**70**(4):557-561

[58] Kelly KN et al. Laparotomy for small-bowel obstruction: First choice or last resort for adhesiolysis? A laparoscopic approach for small-bowel obstruction reduces 30-day complications. Surgical Endoscopy. 2014;**28**(1):65-73

[59] Hackenberg T et al. Laparoscopic versus open surgery for acute adhesive small-bowel obstruction: A propensity score-matched analysis. Scandinavian Journal of Surgery. 2017;**106**(1):28-33

[60] Yao S et al. Does laparoscopic adhesiolysis decrease the risk of recurrent symptoms in small bowel obstruction? A propensity score-matched analysis. Surgical Endoscopy. 2017;**31**(12):5348-5355

[61] Meuleman T et al. Adhesion awareness: A nationwide survey of gynaecologists. European Journal of Obstetrics, Gynecology, and Reproductive Biology. 2013;**169**(2):353-359

[62] Hackethal A et al. Awareness and perception of intra-abdominal adhesions and related consequences: Survey of gynaecologists in German hospitals. European Journal of Obstetrics, Gynecology, and Reproductive Biology. 2010;**150**(2):180-189

[63] ten Broek RP, van den Beukel BA, van Goor H. Comparison of operative notes with real-time observation of adhesiolysis-related complications during surgery. The British Journal of Surgery. 2013;**100**(3):426-432

[64] Kohn LT, Corrigan JM, Donaldson MS. To Err Is Human: Building a Safer Health System. Washington, DC: Institute of Medicine (US) Committee on Quality of Health Care in America; 2000. Available from: https://www.ncbi.nlm.nih.gov/pubmed/25077248

[65] Vonlanthen R et al. The impact of complications on costs of major surgical procedures: A cost analysis of 1200 patients. Annals of Surgery. 2011;**254**(6):907-913

[66] Ramly EP et al. The financial impact of intraoperative adverse events in abdominal surgery. Surgery. 2015;**158**(5):1382-1388

[67] Nandan AR et al. The impact of major intraoperative adverse events on hospital readmissions. American Journal of Surgery. 2017;**213**(1):10-17

[68] Vibert E et al. Arterial lactate concentration at the end of an elective hepatectomy is an early predictor of the

postoperative course and a potential surrogate of intraoperative events. Annals of Surgery. 2015;**262**(5):787-792. discussion 792-3

[69] Kinaci E et al. Intraoperative acidosis is a new predictor for postoperative pancreatic fistula after pancreaticoduodenectomy. Hepatobiliary & Pancreatic Diseases International. 2016;**15**(3):302-309

[70] Parker MC et al. Postoperative adhesions: Ten-year follow-up of 12,584 patients undergoing lower abdominal surgery. Diseases of the Colon and Rectum. 2001;**44**(6):822-829. discussion 829-30

[71] Rosenthal R et al. Definition and classification of intraoperative complications (CLASSIC): Delphi study and pilot evaluation. World Journal of Surgery. 2015;**39**(7):1663-1671

[72] Mavros MN et al. Intraoperative adverse events: Risk adjustment for procedure complexity and presence of adhesions is crucial. Journal of the American College of Surgeons. 2015;**221**(2):345-353

[73] Karamanos E et al. Diabetes mellitus in patients presenting with adhesive small bowel obstruction: Delaying surgical intervention results in worse outcomes. World Journal of Surgery. 2016;**40**(4):863-869

[74] Krielen P et al. Cost-effectiveness of the prevention of adhesions and adhesive small bowel obstruction after colorectal surgery with adhesion barriers: A modelling study. World Journal of Emergency Surgery. 2019;**14**:41

[75] Strik C et al. Risk factors for future repeat abdominal surgery. Langenbeck's Archives of Surgery. 2016;**401**(6):829-837

[76] Weng CH et al. A simple technique for placement of Seprafilm(R)-a sodium hyaluronate/carboxymethylcellulose absorbable barrier-during laparoscopic myomectomy. Journal of Minimally Invasive Gynecology. 2019. Available from: https://pubmed.ncbi.nlm.nih.gov/31877383/

[77] Raimondo D et al. Cellulose absorbable barrier for prevention of de-novo adhesion formation at the time of laparoscopic myomectomy: A systematic review and meta-analysis of randomized controlled trials. European Journal of Obstetrics, Gynecology, and Reproductive Biology. 2019;**245**:107-113

[78] Chaturvedi AA et al. Prevention of postsurgical adhesions using an ultrapure alginate-based gel. The British Journal of Surgery. 2013;**100**(7):904-910

[79] Chaturvedi AA et al. Ultrapure alginate gel reduces adhesion reformation after adhesiolysis. International Journal of Colorectal Disease. 2014;**29**(11):1411-1416

[80] Pilpel Y et al. Metabolic syndrome is a risk factor for post-operative adhesions: Need for novel treatment strategies. Hormone and Metabolic Research. 2019;**51**(1):35-41

[81] Robertson LM et al. Evitar (l-Alanyl-l-glutamine) regulates key signaling molecules in the pathogenesis of postoperative tissue fibrosis. Reproductive Sciences. 2019;**26**(6):724-733

[82] Robertson LM, Rislund DC, Lim HJ, Pierson RA, Tulandi T, Gargiolo AR, et al. A novel therapeutic approach to prevent adhesion: A double blind randomized study (DBRCT) of intraperitoneal L-Alanyl-L-Glutamine (A-G or Evitar™) for the prevention of adhesion in laparoscopic myomectomies. In: Abstract Presentation at 47th Global Congress of Minimally Invasive Gynecology; Las Vegas, Nevada. 2018

Chapter 3

Gallstones Ileus

Giovanni Petracca, Francesco Zappia and Fabrizio Silvaggio

Abstract

The ileus of gallstones is a rare complication of cholelithiasis which occurs in less than 1% of patients and is the cause of 1–4% of cases of obstruction of the small intestine. The pathogenesis involves the formation of a bilioenteric fistula. Abdominal computed tomography (CT) shows pneumobilia, dilated loops of small intestine, and ectopic gallstones that obstruct the intestinal lumen. In literature, enterolithotomy is the most frequently used procedure for the ileum of gallstones. Enterolithotomy plus cholecystectomy and/or fistulectomy are indicated only in selected patients. The clinical signs and symptoms depend on the site of the obstruction and usually include abdominal pain, nausea, and vomiting. The diagnostic test of choice is an abdominal CT scan.

Keywords: gallstone ileus, cholecystoenteric fistula, cholecystitis

1. Introduction

The biliary ileum is defined as a mechanical intestinal obstruction due to the impact of one or more gallstones in the gastrointestinal tract and is a rare complication of cholelithiasis. The term "ileum" is an improper term, since obstruction is a true mechanical phenomenon [1, 2], while gastrointestinal obstruction from gallstones would be an appropriate term. Biliary ileum is not very common and diagnosis and treatment can be problematic.

1.1 Epidemiology

Biliary ileus causes 1–4% of all cases of obstruction of the small intestine. This is 25% in patients over 65 years of age and is responsible for about three of the 10 million admissions to hospital and 15 for about 1 million surgical procedures (0.0015%). It is more common in women than in men with a 5:1 female-to-male ratio.

1.2 Pathophysiology

The biliary ileum is often preceded by an initial episode of acute cholecystitis. Inflammation in the gallbladder and surrounding structures leads to the formation of adhesion. Inflammation and the pressure effect of gallstones causes erosion through the gallbladder wall, leading to the formation of fistulas between the gallbladder and the adiacent portion of the gastrointestinal tract, with further passage of gallstones [3, 4]. Less commonly, a gallstone can enter the duodenum through the common bile duct and through a dilated papilla of Vater [5]. The most frequent fistula occurs between the gallbladder and the duodenum due to their proximity [6–9]. The stomach, small intestine, and transverse portion of the colon may also be involved (**Table 1**) [1–4, 10, 11].

Once inside the duodenal, intestinal, or gastric lumen, gallstones usually proceed distally and can pass spontaneously through the rectum, or they can cause obstruction. Less commonly if the bile stone is in the stomach, proximal migration can occur and the bile stone can be vomited [4]. The size of the gallstones, the site of fistula formation, and the intestinal lumen will determine whether or not intestinal obstruction will occur. Most gallstones less than 2–2.5 cm can pass spontaneously through a normal gastrointestinal tract and will be excreted in the stool without problems [1–4]. Clavien et al. [12] reported that an obstructive gallstone size ranges from 2 to 5 cm. Nakao et al. [6] found that gallstones had sizes ranging from 2 to 10 cm, with an average of 4.3 cm. The obstruction site can be found in any portion of the gastrointestinal tract. If gallstones enter the duodenum, the most common intestinal obstruction will be the terminal ileum and ileocecal valve due to their relatively narrow lumen and potentially less active peristalsis. Less frequently, gallstones obstruct the proximal ileum or jejunum, especially if the gallstones are large enough. Less common positions include the stomach and duodenum (Bouveret syndrome) and colon (**Table 2**) [1, 3, 4, 8, 9, 13].

The presence of diverticula, neoplasms, or intestinal stenoses secondary to Crohn's disease, reduce the size of the lumen and can cause an occlusion of gallstones on the narrowing site [1–3, 14]. Biliary ileum has been reported at anastomosis sites after partial gastrectomy and Billroth II reconstruction and after biliointestinal bypass in two cases [15, 16]. Ischemia can develop at the occlusion site of gallstones due to the pressure generated against the intestinal wall and proximal distension. Necrosis and perforation may occur followed by peritonitis [3]. The presentation of the biliary ileum may be preceded by a history of previous biliary symptoms, with rates ranging between 27 and 80% of patients [7, 12, 13, 17–19]. Acute cholecystitis can be present in 10–30% of patients at the time of intestinal obstruction. Jaundice was found in only 15% of patients or less. Bile symptoms can be absent in up to a third of cases [1–3, 8, 9, 12, 20, 21].

Type of fistula	(%)
Colecystoduodenal	32.5 to 96.5
Colecystogastric	0 to 13.3
Colecystoduodenal	0 to 2,5
Colecystoileal	0 to 2,5
Colecystocolic	0 to 10.9

Table 1.
Frequency of bilio-enteric fistulas in patients with ileus from gallstones.

Place	%
Duodenum	0-10.5
Stomach	0-20
Proximal ileus	0-50
Distal ileus	0-89.5
Colon	0-8.1
Undetermined	0-25

Table 2.
Place range (%).

The biliary ileum can manifest itself as an acute, intermittent, or chronic episode of gastrointestinal obstruction. Nausea, vomiting, cramping abdominal pain, and variable distension are commonly present [1, 3, 8, 12, 13, 20, 22–29]. The intermittent nature of pain and vomiting of the proximal gastrointestinal material, which later becomes dark and fecaloid, is due to partial or total occlusion of gallstones [5, 18]. The character of vomiting depends on the location of the obstruction. When gallstones are in the stomach or upper small intestine, vomiting is mainly gastric in content (becoming fecaloid when the ileum is obstructed). In particular, Bouveret's syndrome presents signs and symptoms of gastric outlet obstruction. Nausea and vomiting were reported in 86% of cases, while abdominal pain or discomfort was reported in 71%. If the bile stone does not completely obstruct the lumen, the presentation will be partially obstructed. Recent weight loss, anorexia, early satiety, and constipation can be reported by the patient. Bouveret syndrome has also been reported to be preceded by bleeding of the upper gastrointestinal tract secondary to duodenal erosion caused by gallstones, with hematemesis and melena, respectively, in 15 and 7% [8, 9, 30, 31]. The physical examination can be nonspecific. Patients are often seriously ill, with signs of dehydration, abdominal distension, and decrease in intestinal peristalsis and obstructive jaundice. Fever, toxicity, and physical signs of peritonitis can be noted if perforation of the intestinal wall occurs. The examination can be completely normal if no obstacles are currently present [1–4, 30].

2. Diagnosis

The symptoms and signs of the biliary ileum are mostly nonspecific [7, 26, 29]. The intermittence of symptoms could also interfere with a correct diagnosis, if the clinical manifestations at the moment correspond to a partial obstruction or a distal migration of the gallstones. Patients usually present 4–8 days after the onset of symptoms, and diagnosis is usually made 3–8 days after the onset of symptoms [1, 2, 29, 32–38]. A high index of suspicion will be useful, particularly in an elderly patient with intestinal obstruction and previous gallstone disease; Bouveret syndrome can be suspected in a patient with gastric outlet obstruction.

2.1 Normal abdominal radiography

Simple abdominal radiographs are of fundamental importance for establishing the diagnosis. In 1941, Rigler et al. [39] described four radiographic signs in the biliary ileum: (1) partial or complete intestinal obstruction; (2) pneumobilia or contrast material in the biliary tree; (3) an aberrant limestone; and (4) changing the position of such gallstones on serial film. The presence of two of the first three signs was considered pathognomonic and was found in 20–50% of cases [1, 2, 20, 37, 38, 40–44]. Although pathognomonic, Rigler's triad ratios range from 0 to 87% [19]. Careful inspection for pneumobilia should be performed, as it is present in most patients with biliary ileus but is sometimes identified only in retrospective observation [20, 37, 38, 41–43]. Pneumobilia can occur following previous biliary surgery or endoscopic interventions. Therefore, clinical evaluation must be taken into account when evaluating this radiological sign [1, 2, 37, 38, 40–44]. In 1978, Balthazar et al. [45] described a fifth sign, which consists of two hydro-plane levels in the upper right quadrant of the abdominal radiography. The medial air fluid level corresponds to the duodenum and the lateral level to the gallbladder. These authors found that this sign was present in 24% of patients at the time of hospitalization. In Bouveret's syndrome, a dilated stomach is expected to be seen on a simple abdominal radiograph due to gastric obstruction [37, 42, 43, 46–49]. Cappell et al. [31], in a review of 64 cases of Bouveret syndrome, found pneumobilia (39%), calcified upper right quadrant mass or gallstones (38%), and gastric distension (23%) as relatively common findings and dilated loops of the intestine (14%).

2.2 Abdominal ultrasound

When the diagnosis is still doubtful, an abdominal ultrasound (US) will be indicated for gallbladder stones, fistula, and gallstones visualization. It can also confirm the presence of choledocholithiasis [1, 2, 50]. The use of ultrasound in combination with abdominal radiography has been recommended to increase the sensitivity of the diagnosis. Ultrasound is more sensitive to the detection of pneumobilia and ectopic gallstones. The combination of abdominal and US radiography increased the sensitivity of the diagnosis of the biliary ileum to 74% [51]. The most frequent findings in Bouveret syndrome are gallstones in the gallbladder (53%), pneumobilia or gallbladder fistula (45%), gallstones in the duodenum (25%), dilated or distended stomach (15%), and a contracted gallbladder (13%) [31, 41, 43, 52, 53].

2.3 Computed tomography

Computed tomography (CT) is considered superior to abdominal radiography or US in the diagnosis of biliary ileum cases, with a sensitivity of up to 93% [47, 51, 54–57]. The detection frequency of Rigler's triad is higher during the CT exam. In a retrospective study by Lassandro et al. [55–58], the Rigler triad was observed in 77.8% of cases by CT, compared to 14.8% with radiographs and 11.1% with the US. Intestinal loop dilation was observed in 92.6% of cases, pneumobilia in 88.9%, ectopic gallstones in 81.5%, hydroaero levels in 37%, and bilio-digestive fistula in 14.8%. Yu et al. [54, 59] conducted a prospective study in which 165 patients with acute small bowel obstruction were evaluated for biliary ileus, with retrospective identification of three diagnostic criteria: (1) small bowel obstruction; (2) ectopic gallstones, both calcified and removed; and (3) abnormal gallbladder with complete air collection, presence of hydro-aircraft levels, or fluid accumulation with irregular wall. The overall sensitivity, specificity, and precision were 93, 100, and 99%, respectively. Rigler's triad was detected only in 36% of cases. These tomographic diagnostic criteria require further prospective validation. Current CT scanners can describe the position of the fistula, gallstones, and gastrointestinal obstruction with greater precision helping in therapeutic decisions [37, 56–58].

2.4 Esophagogastroduodenoscopy

In an 81-case review of Bouveret syndrome [37, 43, 59–62] in which esophagogastroduodenoscopy (EGD) was performed, gastroduodenal obstruction was revealed in all, but visualization of gallstones was only possible in 56 (69%). Among these 56 cases, such gallstones were observed in the duodenal bulb in 51.8%, in the postbulbar duodenum in 28.6%, in the pylorus or in the prepilorum in 17.9%, and in one case the position was not reported. Gallstones were not recognized in 31% of cases because they were deeply embedded in the mucosa. When gallstones are not displayed, the diagnosis should be strongly suspected when the observed mass is hard, convex, smooth, non-friable and non-fleshy, which are all characteristics of a biliary calculus and can improve the sensitivity of the EGD. For such cases, US and CT are the preferred noninvasive diagnostic tests to confirm endoscopic diagnosis, delineate gastroduodenal anatomy, and demonstrate a cholecystoduodenal fistula [27, 31, 52, 53, 63–65].

3. Treatment

The main therapeutic goal is the relief of intestinal obstruction by extraction of gallstones. Hydroelectrolytic imbalances and metabolic disorders due to intestinal obstruction and preexisting comorbidities are common and require management before surgery [1, 2, 14, 29, 31, 52, 53, 66–68].

There is no unanimous consensus on the surgical procedure. Current surgical procedures are: (1) simple enterolithotomy; (2) enterolithotomy, cholecystectomy and closure of the fistula (one-stage procedure); and (3) enterolithotomy with cholecystectomy performed subsequently (two-stage procedure). Intestinal resection is necessary in some cases after performing the enterolithotomy.

Enterolithotomy was the most commonly performed surgical procedure. Through an exploratory laparotomy, the gastrointestinal obstruction site is located. A longitudinal incision is made on the antimesenteric edge proximal to the site of obstruction of the gallstones [12, 24, 66]. Whenever possible, through light manipulation, the bile stone is brought proximally to a non-edematous segment of the intestine. Most of the time, this is not possible due to the degree of impact of gallstones. Enterotomy is performed over the gallstones and extracted. Careful closure of the enterotomy is necessary to avoid narrowing of the intestinal lumen and cross-closure is recommended. Intestinal resection is sometimes required, particularly in the presence of ischemia, perforation, or underlying stenosis [12, 66]. Manual propulsion of gallstones through the ileocecal valve should be reserved for highly selected situations due to the danger of mucosal injury and intestinal perforation [12, 20, 24, 27, 28, 66]. Likewise, attempts to crush gallstones in situ can damage the intestinal wall and should be avoided [20, 27, 66, 69]. Multiple gallstones can generally be extracted through a single incision freeing the intestines and moving smaller gallstones to larger ones. In case of sigmoid obstruction, resection that removes gallstones and underlying stenosis has been recommended [12].

The main long-standing controversy in biliary ileum management is whether surgery should be performed simultaneously with relief of bowel obstruction (one-stage procedure) or later (two-stage procedure).

In 1922, Pybus successfully extracted a limestone blocking the ileum, closed the duodenal fistula, and drained the gallbladder after removing two additional gallstones from it. In 1929, Holz extracted a limestone at the sigmoid level, and after removing a second limestone in the duodenum, he closed the gallbladder fistula and removed the gallbladder. The author recommended this procedure for patients in satisfactory general conditions. In 1957, Welch successfully performed a one-stage surgery in a patient who was well prepared after recurrent intestinal gallstone obstruction. The authors suggested the feasibility of the operation under optimal conditions. In 1965, Berliner et al. [70] reported three similarly managed and mentioned cases that when the patient is adequately hydrated with restored serum electrolytes, it does not represent an operational risk and a one-stage surgical procedure should be considered. The authors recommend considering the one-step procedure in selected cases. The incidence of recurrence commonly cited is 2–5%, but a recurrence of up to 8% has also been reported after only enterolithotomy; half of these new onset events occurred within 30 days [71]. It should be considered that relapse rates of 17–33% have also been reported [12, 72, 73].

The possibility of recurrent cholecystitis and acute cholangitis [12, 70] in patients with unrepaired gallbladder fistulas or retained gallbladder has been highlighted. Acute cholangitis has been reported in 11% of patients with cholecystoduodenal fistula and in 60% with gallbladder colic fistula [12, 52, 53, 67, 68]. With a one-stage procedure, further events related to gallstones are avoided [18].

A potential long-term complication of biliary enteric fistula could be gallbladder cancer. Bossart et al. [74] found an incidence of 15% of gallbladder carcinoma in 57 patients undergoing surgery for these fistulas, compared with 0.8% among all patients with cholecystectomy.

On the other hand, simple enterolithotomy has long been associated with lower mortality [13]. It should be taken into account that the severity of each case affects the outcome of a particular surgical procedure and that mortality is not an absolute consequence of the surgical procedure itself. In the Clavien et al.'s [12] report, when patients were comparable in terms of age, concomitant disease, and APACHE II score, operational mortality and morbidity rates were not significantly different.

In 2003, Doko et al. [75] reported a series of 30 patients with morbidity of 27.3% in patients undergoing enterolithotomy alone and 61.1% for a one-stage procedure. Mortality was 9% after enterolithotomy and 10.5% after a one-stage procedure. The American Society of Anesthesiologists (ASA) scores were similar between the two groups, but operating times were significantly longer for the one-step procedure. Urgent fistula repair was significantly associated with postoperative complications. The authors concluded that enterolithotomy is the procedure of choice, with a one-stage procedure reserved for patients with acute cholecystitis, gallbladder gangrene, or residual gallstones [12].

In 2008, Riaz et al. [76] reported their retrospective experience with 10 patients diagnosed with bileous ileus. The choice of surgical procedure was largely determined by the patient's clinical condition. Five patients underwent enterolithotomy only (group 1), while the remaining five patients underwent cholecystectomy and fistula repair (group 2). In group 1, all patients were hypertensive and diabetic. All patients were hemodynamically unstable, with metabolic acidosis and prerenal azotemia. The ASA score was III or higher in all patients. In group 2, only two patients were hypertensive and all were hemodynamically stable at presentation with an ASA score of II. There was no operational mortality in both groups.

Many patients with biliary ileus are elderly, with comorbidities, in poor general conditions and have a delayed diagnosis, which leads to dehydration, shock, sepsis, or peritonitis. Relief of gastrointestinal obstruction with simple enterolithotomy is the safest procedure for these patients [19, 21].

At laparotomy, examination and careful palpation of the entire intestine, gallbladder, and extrahepatic bile duct is recommended in order to rule out gallstones, bile loss, abscesses, or necrosis [1, 2, 9, 14, 18, 77]. Cholecystectomy and fistula repair reduce the need for reoperation and the incidence of complications related to the persistence of the fistula, including recurrent ileus, cholecystitis, or cholangitis, but are justified only in selected patients who are adequately stabilized in good general condition, with good reserve cardiorespiratory and metabolic, and are able to withstand a more prolonged operation, unless it has been clearly demonstrated that gallstones do not remain in the gallbladder [10, 12, 21, 67, 78, 79].

According to several authors, enterolytictomy alone is the best option for most patients with biliary ileus. The one-step procedure should only be offered to highly selected patients with absolute indications for biliary surgery at the time of presentation and who have been adequately reanimated [6, 7, 13, 21, 29, 31, 52, 53, 67].

The demonstration of gallstones, the appearance of symptoms, or a persistent cholecystointeric fistula indicates the need for cholecystectomy, closure of the fistula, and exploration of the common duct [18]. It has been pointed out that delayed cholecystectomy as a second procedure is clearly justified only in cases of persistence of symptoms [13, 21]. Cholecystectomy and fistula closure are recommended 4–6 weeks later [7, 13, 29, 80]. A 2.94% mortality rate has been reported in this group of patients [25].

4. Morbidity

The most common postoperative complication was wound infection. In 1961, Raiford [5] observed an overall wound infection rate of 75%. Localized peritonitis, respiratory complications, phlebitis, and recurrent obstruction due to residual gallstones and cholangitis have also been observed. Wound infection continues to be the most common complication, with rates of 27 and 42.5%, as reported by Clavien et al. [12] and Rodríguez Hermosa et al. [19], respectively. Several authors have reported no significant differences in postoperative complications between patients treated with enterolithotomy or enterolithotomy, cholecystectomy, and closure of fistulas [12, 21, 67, 80]. The least common complications were wound dehiscence, cardiopulmonary and vascular complications, sepsis, intestinal and biliary fistulas, and urinary tract infections [12, 21, 80].

5. Mortality

Biliary ileum is predominantly a geriatric disease and as many as 80–90% of patients have concomitant medical diseases. Hypertension, diabetes, congestive heart failure, chronic lung disease, and anemia are the most common comorbidities [25]. These associated conditions must be taken into consideration, as they can influence the results of the treatment [1].

Mortality rates were reported up to 44% in the late 1800s, while in the first half of the twentieth century, these rates remained between 40 and 50% [14, 22]. In the 1990s, significant reductions in mortality were observed at 15–18%, at current rates of less than 7% [13, 25]. In particular, simple enterolithotomy has long been associated with a mortality of 11.7% compared to 16.9% for the one-stage procedure (enterolithotomy plus cholecystectomy and fistula closure) [13]. As described by Kirchmayr et al. [79], four main reasons could be responsible for the high number of lethal courses. First of all, the biliary ileum is a disease of the elderly. Second, concomitant diseases such as cardiorespiratory diseases and/or diabetes mellitus are frequent. Third, due to uncommon symptoms, the diagnosis is difficult and an average delay of 4 days from the start of symptoms to hospitalization is reported. Fourth, postoperative recovery is also hampered; age-related complications such as pneumonia or heart failure are more frequent than complications associated with surgery.

The authors noted that fistula closure, performed during the initial procedure, was independently associated with a higher mortality rate than enterolithotomy alone. When intestinal resection was indicated, it was also associated with a higher mortality rate than with enterolithotomy alone. However, if you consider the fact that intestinal resection is not exactly an option but a requirement due to the conditions of the intestinal segment, the mortality for those patients who underwent enterolithotomy alone or intestinal resection is actually 6.53%.

6. Conclusions

Biliary ileum or gastrointestinal obstruction from gallstones accounts for less than 1% of cases of gastrointestinal obstruction, with a higher frequency among the elderly. Computed tomography has proven to be the most accurate diagnostic modality, but validation of diagnostic criteria is required. Surgical relief of the obstruction is the cornerstone of the treatment. Given the high incidence of comorbidity in these patients, a good judgment is needed in the choice of the surgical procedure. Enterolithotomy remains the mainstay of surgical treatment. A one-stage cholecystectomy and fistula repair are justified only in selected patients in good general condition and adequately stabilized preoperatively. Two-stage surgery is an option for patients with persistent symptoms after an enterolithotomy. Extensive prospective studies of laparoscopic and endoscopic guided procedures are planned.

Author details

Giovanni Petracca*, Francesco Zappia and Fabrizio Silvaggio
Ospedale "G. Jazzolino" – Vibo Valentia, Azienda Sanitaria Provinciale di Vibo Valentia, Vibo Valentia, Italy

*Address all correspondence to: doc37@virgilio.it

References

[1] Abou-Saif A, Al-Kawas FH. Complications of gallstone disease: Mirizzi syndrome, cholecystocholedochal fistula, and gallstone ileus. The American Journal of Gastroenterology. 2002;**97**:249-254

[2] Martin F. Intestinal obstruction due to gall-stones: With report of three successful cases. Annals of Surgery. 1912;**55**:725-743

[3] Fox PF. Planning the operation for cholecystoenteric fistula with gallstone ileus. The Surgical Clinics of North America. 1970;**50**:93-102

[4] VanLandingham SB, Broders CW. Gallstone ileus. The Surgical Clinics of North America. 1982;**62**:241-247

[5] Raiford TS. Intestinal obstruction due to gallstones. (Gallstone ileus). Annals of Surgery. 1961;**153**:830-838

[6] Nakao A, Okamoto Y, Sunami M, Fujita T, Tsuji T. The oldest patient with gallstone ileus: Report of a case and review of 176 cases in Japan. The Kurume Medical Journal. 2008;**55**:29-33

[7] Ayantunde AA, Agrawal A. Gallstone ileus: diagnosis and management. World Journal of Surgery. 2007;**31**:1292-1297

[8] Masannat Y, Masannat Y, Shatnawei A. Gallstone ileus: A review. Mount Sinai Journal of Medicine. 2006;**73**:1132-1134

[9] Beltran MA, Csendes A. Mirizzi syndrome and gallstone ileus: An unusual presentation of gallstone disease. Journal of Gastrointestinal Surgery. 2005;**9**:686-689

[10] Ploneda-Valencia CF, Gallo-Morales M, Rinchon C, Navarro-Muñiz E, Bautista-López CA, de la Cerda-Trujillo LF, et al. Gallstone ileus: An overview of the literature. Revista de Gastroenterología de México. 2017;**82**(3):248-254. DOI: 10.1016/j.rgmx.2016.07.006

[11] Abbasi S-U-N, Khan DB, Khandwala K, Raza R, Memon WA. Cholecystocolonic fistula. Case Reports. 2019;**11**(6):e4874

[12] Clavien PA, Richon J, Burgan S, Rohner A. Gallstone ileus. The British Journal of Surgery. 1990;**77**:737-742

[13] Reisner RM, Cohen JR. Gallstone ileus: A review of 1001 reported cases. The American Surgeon. 1994;**60**:441-446

[14] Rogers FA, Carter R. Gallstone intestinal obstruction. California Medicine. 1958;**88**:140-143

[15] Dias AR, Lopes RI. Biliary stone causing afferent loop syndrome and pancreatitis. World Journal of Gastroenterology. 2006;**12**:6229-6231

[16] Micheletto G, Danelli P, Morandi A, Panizzo V, Montorsi M. Gallstone ileus after biliointestinal bypass: Report of two cases. Journal of Gastrointestinal Surgery. 2013;**17**:2162-2165

[17] Mondragón Sánchez A, Berrones Stringel G, Tort Martínez A, Soberanes Fernández C, Domínguez Camacho L, Mondragón Sánchez R. Surgical management of gallstone ileus: Fourteen year experience. Revista de Gastroenterología de México. 2005;**70**:44-49

[18] Warshaw AL, Bartlett MK. Choice of operation for gallstone intestinal obstruction. Annals of Surgery. 1966;**164**:1051-1055

[19] Rodríguez Hermosa JI, Codina Cazador A, Gironès Vilà J, Roig García J, Figa Francesch M, Acero Fernández D. Gallstone ileus: Results of analysis of a

series of 40 patients. Gastroenterología y Hepatología. 2001;**24**:489-494

[20] Luu MB, Deziel DJ. Unusual complications of gallstones. The Surgical Clinics of North America. 2014;**94**:377-394

[21] Rodríguez-Sanjuán JC, Casado F, Fernández MJ, Morales DJ, Naranjo A. Cholecystectomy and fistula closure versus enterolithotomy alone in gallstone ileus. The British Journal of Surgery. 1997;**84**:634-637

[22] Courvoisier LG. Casuistisch-statistische Beitrage zur Pathologic und Chirurgie der gallenwege. XII Leipzig: FCW Vogel; 1890

[23] Bouveret L. Stenose du pylore adherent a la vesicule calculeuse. Revolution Medicines. 1896;**16**:1-16

[24] Kurtz RJ, Heimann TM, Beck AR, Kurtz AB. Patterns of treatment of gallstone ileus over a 45-year period. The American Journal of Gastroenterology. 1985;**80**:95-98

[25] Halabi WJ, Kang CY, Ketana N, Lafaro KJ, Nguyen VQ, Stamos MJ, et al. Surgery for gallstone ileus: A nationwide comparison of trends and outcomes. Annals of Surgery. 2014;**259**:329-335

[26] Kasahara Y, Umemura H, Shiraha S, Kuyama T, Sakata K, Kubota H. Gallstone ileus. Review of 112 patients in the Japanese literature. American Journal of Surgery. 1980;**140**:437-440

[27] Habib E, Elhadad A. Digestive complications of gallstones lost during laparoscopic cholecystectomy. HPB: The Official Journal of the International Hepato Pancreato Biliary Association. 2003;**5**:118-122

[28] Zehetner J, Shamiyeh A, Wayand W. Lost gallstones in laparoscopic cholecystectomy: All possible complications. American Journal of Surgery. 2007;**193**:73-78

[29] Zaliekas J, Munson JL. Complications of gallstones: The Mirizzi syndrome, gallstone ileus, gallstone pancreatitis, complications of "lost" gallstones. The Surgical Clinics of North America. 2008;**88**:1345-1368

[30] Koulaouzidis A, Moschos J. Bouveret's syndrome. Narrative review. Annals of Hepatology. 2007;**6**:89-91

[31] Cappell MS, Davis M. Characterization of Bouveret's syndrome: A comprehensive review of 128 cases. The American Journal of Gastroenterology. 2006;**101**:2139-2146

[32] Jakubauskas M, Luksaite R, Sileikis A, Strupas I, Poskus T. Gallstone ileus: Management and clinical outeomes. Medicina. 2019;**55**(9):598

[33] De Monti M, Cestaro G, Alkayyali S, Galafassi J, Fasolini F. Gallstone ileus: A possible cause of bowel obstruction in thè elderly population. International Journal of Surgery Case Report. 2018;**43**:18-23

[34] Al-Mudares S, Kurer M, Koshy RM, El-Menyar A. An unusual presentation of gallstone ileus: A red-herring or missed diagnosis. American Journal of Case Reports. 2016;**17**:301

[35] Ramirez-Ramirez MM, Villanueva-Saenz E, Zubieta-Ófarril G. Rigler's triad in gallstone ileus: A rare form of bowel obstruction. Revista di Gastroenterología de México. 2016;**81**(2):103-104

[36] Sertkaya M, Emre A, Akbulut S, Vicdan H, Şanh AN. A typical gallstone ileus: Clinical, radiological and operational findings. Turkish Journal of Gastroenterology 2019; 30: 377-380

[37] Aldo IO, Lorenzo M, Olgerta L, Alberto C, Licia U, Melchiore G. Rolling

in thè deep: Imaging findings and diagnostic pearls in gallstone. Surgery Research and Practice. 2020;**1421753**

[38] Shovkat Ahmad Mir, Zeiad Hussain, Christine Ann Davey, Glenn Vincent Miller, Srinivas Chintapatla. Management and outcome of recurrent gallstone ileus: A systematic review. World Journal of Gastrointestinal Surgery 2015;7(8):152-159.

[39] Rigler LG, Borman CN, Noble JF. Gallstone obstruction: Pathogenesis and roentgen manifestations. Journal of the American Medical Association. 1941;**117**:1753-1759

[40] Haddad FG, Mansour W, Mansour J, Deeb L. From Bouveret's syndrome to gallstone ileus: The journey of a migrating stone! 1 Cureus. 2018;**10**(3):e2370

[41] Rotaru MI, Necula AH, Caraiani CN, Badea AF, Tantau MV, Badea RI. Point-of-care ultrasound in management of Gallstone ileus - A case report. Medical Ultrasonography. 2019;**21**(2):197-199

[42] Saran S, Malik S, Kharbanda A, Sharma Y. Pneumobilia with multiple air-fluid levels on abdominal radiography: A clincher. Annals of African Medicine. 2019;**18**(2):115-116

[43] Ferhatoğlu MF, Kartal A. Bouveret's syndrome: A case-based review, clinical presentation, diagnostics and treatment approaches. SiSli Etfal Hastanesi Tip Bulteni. 2020;**54**(1):1-7

[44] Morosin T, De Robles MSB, Putnis S. Gallstone ileus: An unusual cause of intestinal obstruction. Cureus. 2020;**12**(3):e7284

[45] Balthazar EJ, Schechter LS. Air in gallbladder: A frequent finding in gallstone ileus. AJR. American Journal of Roentgenology. 1978;**131**:219-222

[46] Liew V, Layani L, Speakman D. Bouveret's syndrome in Melbourne. ANZ Journal of Surgery. 2002;**72**:161-163

[47] Brennan GB, Rosenberg RD, Arora S. Bouveret syndrome. Radiographics. 2004;**24**:1171-1175

[48] Chang L, Chang M, Chang HM, Chang AI, Chang F. Clinical and radiological diagnosis of gallstone ileus. Emergency Radiology. 2018;**25**:189-196. DOI: 10.1007/s10140-017-1568-5

[49] Tahashi K, Kashimura H, Konno N, Nakagawa M, Kawahara Y, Munakata A, et al. Gallstone ileus with spontaneous evacuation: A case report. Journal of General and Family Medicine. 2018;**19**(5):173-175

[50] Lasson A, Lorén I, Nilsson A, Nirhov N, Nilsson P. Ultrasonography in gallstone ileus: A diagnostic challenge. The European Journal of Surgery. 1995;**161**:259-263

[51] Ripollés T, Miguel-Dasit A, Errando J, Morote V, Gómez-Abril SA, Richart J. Gallstone ileus: Increased diagnostic sensitivity by combining plain film and ultrasound. Abdominal Imaging. 2001;**26**:401-405

[52] Cooperman AM, Dickson ER, ReMine WH. Changing concepts in the surgical treatment of gallstone ileus: A review of 15 cases with emphasis on diagnosis and treatment. Annals of Surgery. 1968;**167**:377-383

[53] de Alencastro MC, Cardoso KT, Mendes CA, Boteon YL, de Carvalho RB, Fraga GP. Acute intestinal obstruction due to gallstone ileus. Revista do Colégio Brasileiro de Cirurgiões. 2013;**40**:275-280

[54] Yu CY, Lin CC, Shyu RY, Hsieh CB, Wu HS, Tyan YS, et al. Value of CT in the diagnosis and management of gallstone ileus. World Journal of Gastroenterology. 2005;**11**:2142-2147

[55] Lassandro F, Gagliardi N, Scuderi M, Pinto A, Gatta G, Mazzeo R. Gallstone ileus analysis of radiological findings in 27 patients. European Journal of Radiology. 2004;**50**:23-29

[56] Lassandro F, Romano S, Ragozzino A, Rossi G, Valente T, Ferrara I, et al. Role of helical CT in diagnosis of gallstone ileus and related conditions. AJR. American Journal of Roentgenology. 2005;**185**:1159-1165

[57] Balthazar EJ, George W. Holmes lecture. CT of small-bowel obstruction. AJR. American Journal of Roentgenology. 1994;**162**:255-261

[58] Pickhardt PJ, Friedland JA, Hruza DS, Fisher AJ. Case report. CT, MR cholangiopancreatography, and endoscopy findings in Bouveret's syndrome. AJR. American Journal of Roentgenology. 2003;**180**:1033-1035

[59] Bruni SG, Pickup M, Thorpe D. Bouveret's syndrome-a rare form of gallstone ileus causing death: Appearance on post-mortem CT and MRI. BJR. 2017;**3**(3):20170032

[60] Caldwell KM, Lee SJ, Leggett PL, Bajwa KS, Mehta SS, Shah SIC. Bouveret syndrome: Current management strategies. Clinical and Experimental Gastroenterology. 2018;**11**:69-75

[61] Yu Y-B, Song Y, Xu J-B, Qi F-Z. Bouveret's syndrome: A rare presentation of gastric outlet obstruction. Experimental and Therapeutic Medicine. 2019;**17**(3):1813-1816

[62] Evola G, Caramma S, Caruso G, Dapri G, Evola FR, Reina C, et al. Bouveret's syndrome as a rare complication of Cholelithiasis: Disputes in current management and report of two cases. Surgical Case Reports. 2020;**71**:315-318

[63] Halter F, Bangerter U, Gigon JP, Pusterla C. Gallstone ileus after endoscopic sphincterotomy. Endoscopy. 1981;**13**:88-89

[64] Chavalitdhamrong D, Donepudi S, Pu L, Draganov PV. Uncommon and rarely reported adverse events of endoscopic retrograde cholangiopancreatography. Digestive Endoscopy. 2014;**26**:15-22

[65] Yamauchi Y, Wakui N, Asai Y, Dan N, Takeda Y, Ueki N, et al. Gallstone ileus following endoscopic stone extraction. Case Reports in Gastrointestinal Medicine. 2014;**2014**:271571

[66] Deckoff SL. Gallstone ileus; a report of 12 cases. Annals of Surgery. 1955;**142**:52-65

[67] Martínez Ramos D, Daroca José JM, Escrig Sos J, Paiva Coronel G, Alcalde Sánchez M, Salvador Sanchís JL. Gallstone ileus: Management options and results on a series of 40 patients. Revista Española de Enfermedades Digestivas. 2009;**101**:117-120

[68] Yakan S, Engin O, Tekeli T, Calik B, Deneçli AG, Coker A, et al. Gallstone ileus as an unexpected complication of cholelithiasis: Diagnostic difficulties and treatment. Ulusal Travma ve Acil Cerrahi Dergisi. 2010;**16**:344-348

[69] Aguilar-Espinosa F, Maza-Sánchez R, Vargas-Solís F, Guerrero-MartínezGA,Medina-ReyesJL, Flores-Quiroz PI. Cholecystoduodenal fistula, an infrequent complication of Cholelithiasis: Our experience in its surgical management. Revista de Gastroenterología de México. 2017;**82**(4):287-295. DOI: 10.1016/j.rgmx.2016.10.010

[70] Berliner SD, Burson LC. One-stage repair for cholecyst-duodenal fistula and gallstone ileus. Archives of Surgery. 1965;**90**:313-316

[71] Doogue MP, Choong CK, Frizelle FA. Recurrent gallstone ileus: Underestimated. The Australian and New Zealand Journal of Surgery. 1998;**68**:755-756

[72] Kirkland KC, Croce EJ. Gallstone intestinal obstruction. A review of the literature and presentation of 12 cases, including 3 recurrences. Journal of the American Medical Association. 1961;**176**:494-497

[73] Ravikumar R, Williams JG. The operative management of gallstone ileus. Annals of the Royal College of Surgeons of England. 2010;**92**:279-281

[74] Bossart PA, Patterson AH, Zintel HA. Carcinoma of the gallbladder. A report of seventy-six cases. American Journal of Surgery. 1962;**103**:366-369

[75] Doko M, Zovak M, Kopljar M, Glavan E, Ljubicic N, Hochstädter H. Comparison of surgical treatments of gallstone ileus: Preliminary report. World Journal of Surgery. 2003;**27**:400-404

[76] Riaz N, Khan MR, Tayeb M. Gallstone ileus: Retrospective review of a single centre's experience using two surgical procedures. Singapore Medical Journal. 2008;**49**:624-626

[77] Fiddian RV. Gall-stone ileus. Recurrences and multiple stones. Postgraduate Medical Journal. 1959;**35**:673-676

[78] Nuño-Guzmán CM, Arróniz-Jáuregui J, Moreno-Pérez PA, Chávez-Solís EA, Esparza-Arias N, Hernández-González CI. Gallstone ileus: One-stage surgery in a patient with intermittent obstruction. World Journal of Gastrointestinal Surgery. 2010;**2**:172-176

[79] Kirchmayr W, Mühlmann G, Zitt M, Bodner J, Weiss H, Klaus A. Gallstone ileus: rare and still controversial. ANZ Journal of Surgery. 2005;**75**:234-238

[80] Tan YM, Wong WK, Ooi LL. A comparison of two surgical strategies for the emergency treatment of gallstone ileus. Singapore Medical Journal. 2004;**45**:69-72

Chapter 4

Foreign Bodies and Bowel Obstructions

Jessica Elizabeth Taylor and Devin Clegg

Abstract

Foreign body ingestion most commonly occurs in the pediatric population, with approximately 80–90% of objects passing spontaneously in individuals who are evaluated by medical professionals. Objects may be lodged in a variety of anatomic locations. Only about 10% of foreign bodies progress past the stomach. Of the 10–20% of objects that fail to pass, less than 1% requires surgical intervention. Small bowel obstructions are a rare presentation of foreign body ingestions. There are case reports, guidelines, and retrospective reviews in the literature regarding the management of ingested foreign bodies. In patients who do not have spontaneous passage of foreign bodies, endoscopic and surgical techniques have been utilized for successful retrieval. The timing and indication for endoscopic intervention is dependent upon several factors, including the type and location of the foreign body and is also contingent upon patient symptoms. Numerous case reports and studies describe the successful endoscopic removal of foreign bodies in the upper and lower gastrointestinal tract. Although the type and location of an ingested object is critical for determining the success of endoscopic intervention, the patient's clinical exam and stability is also an aspect to consider when deciding on management of bowel obstructions caused by foreign bodies.

Keywords: foreign body, ingestion, obstruction, intestine, bowel

1. Introduction

Foreign body ingestion encompasses a wide range of objects. Most often, the patients that have ingested a foreign body are in the pediatric population, which can lead to its own challenges in management. In adults, there is even less literature that discusses foreign body ingestion and outcomes.

Foreign bodies can become lodged in various areas of the upper and lower gastrointestinal tracts. There are specific characteristics of objects and certain anatomic and physiologic regions of the gastrointestinal tract that create unique problems regarding management of the ingested foreign body. As is demonstrated in the pediatric literature, an algorithmic approach should be utilized to manage adults who have ingested an object. This approach includes systematic evaluation and work-up, determining appropriate management based on the clinical evaluation, and ultimately addressing complications as they may arise during the management process.

2. Evaluation and work-up

2.1 Clinical history

A very important aspect in the evaluation of foreign body ingestion is obtaining an accurate history. Whether the patient is pediatric or adult, if there was a witness to the ingestion, then determining the exact foreign body and its characteristics will be easier to determine. Adult ingestions, like pediatric, may be intentional or unintentional. Most adult foreign body ingestions occur in patients with developmental delay, elderly individuals, and prisoners seeking a secondary gain [1]. In these patients obtaining a history may be more challenging. The primary information that needs to be gathered during the history of present illness is type of foreign body, when it was ingested, and the onset of any associated symptoms [1]. When the clinician can determine characteristics about the type of foreign body, then it makes the decision on whether to pursue further diagnostic work-up less challenging.

Foreign bodies may be classified into several categories. **Table 1** lists the categories most often ingested. In the pediatric population, household objects are the most commonly ingested, which include coins, toys, jewelry, magnets, and batteries [1]. Following foreign body ingestion, children may present with symptoms immediately. In adults, objects such as partial dentures, razor blades, and toothbrushes have been reported as being ingested [2]. The size of the ingested objects impacts if these foreign bodies will become lodged and unable to pass through the gastrointestinal tract; although, it is reported in the literature that 80–90% of ingested foreign bodies pass spontaneously [3].

The European Society of Gastrointestinal Endoscopy (ESGE) Clinical Guidelines recommend that diagnostic evaluation be considered based on the patient's history and symptoms. The symptoms that would indicate the presence of an esophageal foreign body include dysphagia, odynophagia, or chest pain. Other symptoms that may also be present include sore throat and vomiting. If the foreign body located in the esophagus is large, it may also cause respiratory symptoms due to compression on the trachea [1]. When the ingested foreign body has migrated through the esophagus patients may not report any symptoms.

Aspects of the patient's history that may be underappreciated include past medical problems and surgical procedures. When taking an adequate history, it is important to elucidate whether the patient has a history of inflammatory bowel disease or known malignancies that could impact the passage of the foreign body. Disease processes such as Crohn's or colon cancer could cause stricturing or narrowing in the gastrointestinal tract which may predispose the ingested foreign body to cause an obstruction or other complication. The past surgical history is also important to document, as past abdominal procedures could have altered the anatomy and created additional areas of narrowing which may inhibit the object from passing without complication. After obtaining a thorough history from the patient or other witnesses, then it is appropriate to proceed to physical examination.

Ingested foreign body classifications
Blunt
Sharp
Long

Table 1.
Foreign body classifications.

2.2 Physical examination

The importance of the physical examination should not be underestimated when evaluating a patient with a suspected foreign body ingestion. Although the esophagus is the most common location for a foreign body to become lodged, once it passes into the stomach there are anatomic areas where it has a higher risk of causing obvious signs on physical examination. If the object fails to pass through the esophagus, there may be obvious findings on physical exam such as choking, stridor, or dyspnea, which may be due to aspiration of saliva [1]. In contrast, if the object becomes lodged in the stomach, then the patient may present with abdominal tenderness and distension with associated symptoms of nausea and vomiting. The small intestine, specifically at the ileocecal valve, is another location where a foreign body may cause physical exam findings consistent with obstruction.

The gastrointestinal tract has several anatomic areas of narrowing, which are listed in **Table 2**. One physiological angulation that has been reported to cause difficulty in allowing foreign bodies to pass is the duodenal sweep. If an object is lodged in one of these areas pain may be present on physical exam or as a presenting symptom.

The areas of interest with regards to intestinal obstructions or complications include the ileocecal valve, anus, and duodenal sweep. If the patient has undergone prior operative procedures, in addition to the anatomic areas of narrowing, adhesions or alterations in intestinal anatomy may impact the passage of an ingested foreign body. Examining the abdomen for previous scars and evidence of surgical procedures should be carefully performed, especially in patients who are unable to communicate their past medical and surgical histories.

In patients who present with possible complications related to foreign body ingestion, physical exam findings may be more concerning. Patients with a perforation due to ingested foreign body may have vitals and exam findings which include tachycardia, fever, and peritonitis [1]. If the decision is made to admit and observe a patient who has ingested a foreign body, then monitoring vitals and serial exams becomes an important part in management.

2.3 Diagnostic work-up

Following a thorough history and physical examination, diagnostic work-up should be initiated based on the information gathered from the patient. The diagnostic work-up can include labs and imaging. The imaging techniques discussed in the literature ranges from plain X-rays to CT scans.

Anatomic areas of narrowing in gastrointestinal tract
Upper esophageal sphincter
Aortic arch
Left main stem bronchus
Lower esophageal sphincter
Pylorus
Ileocecal valve
Anus

Table 2.
Anatomic narrowing of GI tract.

Once it is established that a patient has ingested a foreign body, the initial imaging recommended by ESGE is plain X-ray evaluation of the neck, chest, or abdomen depending on the information obtained from the history. The purpose of the imaging is to determine several key pieces of information. Plain films are useful in establishing, initially, the actual presence of a foreign body. Second, X-rays can also provide an estimation as to the size and location. If multiple objects are suspected of being ingested, such as magnets, then the imaging can also help determine the number of foreign bodies [1]. Additionally, complications such perforation or obstruction may also be detected on initial plain films.

Other reports in the literature have discussed using serial X-rays to evaluate passage of objects, specifically magnets in the pediatric population. The protocol suggested by the North American Societies of Pediatric Gastroenterology, Hepatology, and Nutrition includes obtaining serial X-rays every 4–6 hours to monitor for progression [4]. Although obtaining serial abdominal films is considered a diagnostic study, it is also concurrently a part of the non-operative management of foreign body ingestion.

Despite plain radiographs being recommended as the initial diagnostic imaging, there is a reported false-negative rate of 47% [1]. Common objects that are not easily visualized on X-rays include wood, chicken bones, glass, and plastic [1]. If an adequate history supports the ingestion of an object that is difficult to visualize on initial work-up, then further imaging should be performed. Most literature supports that if a complication of foreign body ingestion is suspected, such as perforation or obstruction, then CT scan is the imaging of choice to perform for further evaluation [1].

Figure 1 shows a CT scan obtained in the emergency department on a patient with mental disability and history of PICA. The patient was unable to provide a

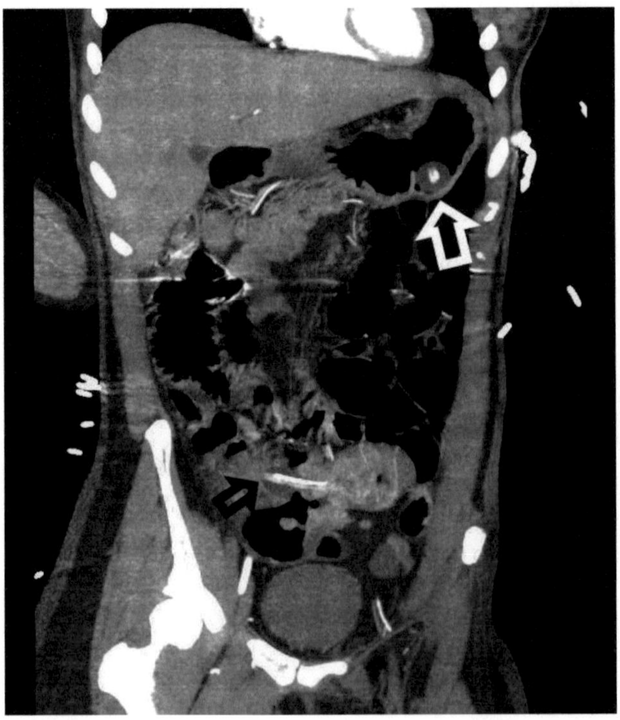

Figure 1.
CT scan demonstrating small bowel obstruction caused by foreign body. Black arrow represents foreign body and white arrow demonstrates patient's functional gastrostomy tube.

history, but per her caregivers she was noted to have increasing abdominal distension and blood coming from her ostomy. Review of the CT scan demonstrated a foreign body causing an obstruction at the ileocecal valve.

Some literature in the pediatric population supports the use of ultrasound in evaluating foreign bodies in the gastrointestinal tract. One published case series showed that different sizes and types of ingested objects can be visualized using point-of-care ultrasound. Other parts of the study demonstrated that ultrasound can also be used to locate foreign bodies within the gastrointestinal tract as well as look for signs of bowel obstruction. Overall, the literature is lacking with regards to ultrasound use in foreign body ingestion, and further studies should be conducted to determine if it is an appropriate substitute for X-ray imaging when evaluating ingested foreign bodies [5].

3. Management

3.1 Important considerations

The literature describing intestinal obstructions due to foreign bodies is replete with case reports, citing many different strategies that are unique based on patient, location, time course and object type, as well as facility resources. More than 100,000 foreign body ingestions are reported each year, with estimated mortality rates around 3% [6]. As previously mentioned, foreign body ingestion is most common in the pediatric population with the peak incidence between ages 6 months and 6 years [7]. This can also be encountered frequently by the general surgeon in the adult population. While the management of foreign bodies is generally well described when located in the upper gastrointestinal (GI) tract, those that pass beyond the gastroesophageal junction and eventually into the lower GI tract are less well documented. While considering the management of these patients, you must consider that between 80 and 95% of objects that traverse the gastroesophageal junction pass through the gastrointestinal tract without further complication, in both pediatrics and adults [6, 8]. Ingestions of foreign bodies or impacted food can lead to the need for emergency endoscopic intervention in 10–20% of cases, with only about 10% of foreign bodies progressing past the stomach, and only 1% requiring surgical intervention [6, 9]. While up to 80% of total foreign body ingestions occur in pediatric patients, in the adult population true foreign body ingestion of nonfood objects more commonly occurs in those with psychiatric illnesses and developmental delay [10].

3.2 Initial management

With all foreign body ingestions, or in rare cases, migrations, the clinician must decide whether the intervention is warranted, the degree of urgency needed, and by what approach. Initial management of foreign body ingestion is first concerned with discerning signs and symptoms of airway compression as these patients may need a definitive airway with endotracheal intubation or other adjuncts. Asymptomatic patients can often describe what or how the object or foreign body was ingested which will aid in determining course of treatment. Patients who have passed the foreign object beyond the gastroesophageal junction or into the distal gastrointestinal tract may present with signs and symptoms of obstruction or perforation. This includes abdominal pain, fever, vomiting or peritonitis [8]. Patients presenting with these symptoms often undergo imaging initially and in rare cases, can present with obstruction or perforation secondary to previously placed surgical materials [6, 11, 12]. Abdominal plain films can be used to follow most radiopaque objects, but CT scan is recommended to delineate more detail. Patients with known foreign body ingestion can be expectantly managed with serial abdominal exams or serial imaging as most foreign bodies that have passed through the esophagus will be excreted without further injury. This is true even for sharp-pointed objects, despite an increased risk of perforation [7].

Impaction, perforation, or obstruction occurs most often at areas of acute angulation or narrowing such as the level of the cricopharyngeus muscle and the ileocecal valve. Other areas of concern, specifically with longer shaped objects, include the pylorus and duodenal c-loop [6]. Patients with prior GI tract surgery or congenitally malformed guts are at increased risk for obstruction and perforation and should be considered for intervention with any change in abdominal exam or imaging [7]. In addition to the signs and symptoms of perforation or obstruction, persistence of an asymptomatic foreign body in the stomach can be a relative indication for endoscopic retrieval, and those lodged distal to the stomach in a fixed persistent location for longer than 1 week may warrant operative intervention [8]. It has been suggested that the time required to excrete a foreign body is between 4 and 6 days, and rarely up to 4 weeks, with retention time in the duodenum being particularly important. If the object is retained in the duodenum for longer than 7 days, it has been shown to have an increased risk of perforation [9]. Gastrointestinal perforation requires emergent operative intervention, with bowel perforation often managed with an open approach, but can be considered for a laparoscopic approach depending on surgeon comfort and availability.

3.3 Endoscopic management

Urgent endoscopic management is often necessary when foreign body ingestion results in impaction within the esophagus, especially when the object is sharp or a button battery. It is also required to prevent aspiration when the foreign object or food bolus impaction creates a high-grade obstruction causing difficulty in managing secretions. Rigid and flexible esophagoscopy are both effective and safe methods of intervention for the removal of esophageal foreign bodies [7]. As rigid esophagoscopy requires general anesthesia, use of a flexible scope may be more feasible in certain situations.

Foreign objects that traverse the pylorus and are located in the distal gastrointestinal tract can still be retrieved endoscopically in certain situations. Single and double-balloon enteroscopy (DBE) can access the small intestine and is emerging as a reliable method of retrieval based on operator comfort and availability [9]. Accessories for the treatment of foreign bodies such as hoods, baskets and forceps have been designed for enteroscopes. Case reports have described the successful retrieval of retained video capsules [3, 12]. Asymptomatic patients are more likely to be candidates for endoscopic management, but case reports have described successful retrieval of retained objects at risk for obstruction or perforation [3]. As DBE is minimally invasive, it theoretically should decrease the length of hospitalization when compared with laparotomy and laparoscopy, although a study has not been specifically performed for this purpose.

The patient whose CT scan was shown in **Figure 1** underwent colonoscopy in an attempt to obtain the foreign body. **Figure 2** demonstrates the endoscopic retrieval of a gastrostomy tube that was causing an obstruction at the terminal ileum. The patient had ingested the feeding tube, and it migrated through the gastrointestinal tract until becoming lodged in the small bowel.

Other forms of lower endoscopy can also be considered based on object location and patient characteristics and include the use of a colonoscope. Endoscopic guidelines have been published more extensively but pertain particularly to the

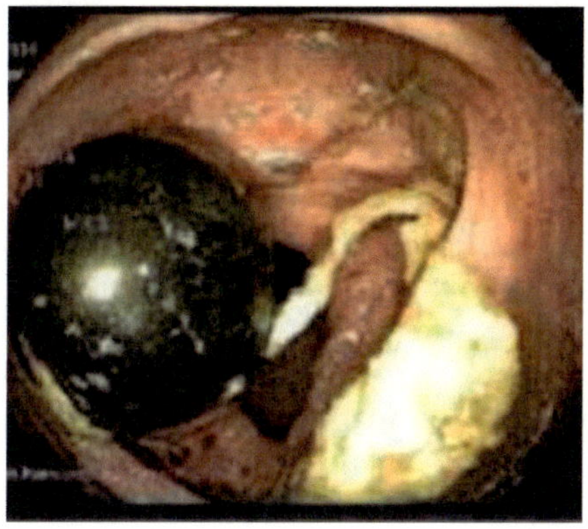

Figure 2.
Colonoscopy showing retrieval of foreign body.

management of the upper gastrointestinal tract, and in the pediatric population [3, 7, 8, 13]. Guidelines for the management of foreign bodies in the lower gastrointestinal tract likely require more data and studies to be performed prior to formal recommendations. At this time, management is trending strongly towards the use of endoscopy for stable patients, while unstable patients or those at high-risk for perforation are managed operatively.

3.4 Surgical management

Surgical management is often reserved for patients that present emergently with bowel obstruction, abscess formation, or perforation secondary to the foreign body ingestion. These patients have traditionally undergone open procedures as a first choice, but with advances in technique and availability, laparoscopic approaches are being more commonly reported as a successful alternative.

3.5 Laparoscopic management

Laparoscopy is an important method to consider when approaching the management of patients with retained foreign objects in the distal gastrointestinal tract. The trend towards minimally invasive surgery has been supported by decreased length of hospitalization and a lower rate of complication in abdominal surgery when compared to laparotomy. The use of this method largely depends on surgeon comfort, training and availability, as many facilities defer to laparotomy for management due to these limiting factors.

Most of the information on laparoscopic management of intestinal obstructions related to foreign body ingestion is anecdotal, with few studies being performed to date. A five-patient case series from Chia et al. reported successful management with laparoscopy after failed endoscopy. Three of five patients had abscess formation, with two patients complicated by perforation. All five had successful retrieval of the foreign body and primary repair of the bowel with intracorporeal suturing, as well as successful deroofing and drainage of the abscesses if needed [14]. Other case reports have reported similar methods and results, with some describing enterotomy and intracorporeal repair after retrieval [11, 15].

It is important to note, that with any surgical intervention performed, it is recommended that any potentially involved bowel be visualized for perforation or injury. As with all bowel injuries, if greater than 50% of its circumference, resection and anastomosis is recommended.

3.6 Open surgical management

Laparotomy is still recommended for management of the unstable patient with suspected or confirmed perforation or obstruction that is threatening life or bowel. This presentation secondary to foreign body obstruction is rare, but it is important to consider. As the management trend has shifted towards minimally invasive, with endoscopic management often attempted first and laparoscopy considered if available, open surgical management is often reserved for emergency or for those facilities that do not have the resources the previously mentioned approaches [8, 9, 16, 17]. As with the laparoscopic management, the area of obstruction, perforation or abscess formation should be localized and an enterotomy made for retrieval. If the bowel is viable and can be repaired primarily this is recommended. If bowel injury is greater than 50% of its circumference, resection and anastomosis is recommended. If the patient is unstable and requires further resuscitation, or the abdomen is grossly contaminated, damage control surgery is always a consideration with the patient left in discontinuity after the object has been removed and further contamination has been controlled.

Intervention upon retained foreign object is largely dependent on the characteristics of the patient, the object, the time course and the presentation, as well as the resources available at the facility. As the majority of foreign objects pass without injury through the gastrointestinal tract, it is relatively rare for ingestion to result in surgical intervention. A clear trend towards the most minimally invasive approach has been forming, and we anticipate that the future guidelines will reflect this. The basic principles of bowel obstruction and perforation are still the most important factors to consider when planning your method of management and should be adhered to.

4. Complications

4.1 Perforation

Foreign body ingestion resulting in perforation is a rare but dreaded complication. It is reported to occur following only 1% of foreign body ingestions [18]. Some studies in the literature report that the average time from ingestion to evaluation at a medical facility was 10.4 ± 9.3 days with a wide range of 3 to 60 days [19]. The most common presenting symptom at the time of presentation is abdominal pain, with many patients having peritonitis on exam. Once a diagnosis of perforation is suspected, operative exploration is warranted. The most common locations found intra-operatively are the distal ileum and colon. Other less common locations are the duodenum and jejunum. Reports in the literature support that longer objects often result in more proximal intestinal perforation at the second and third portion of the duodenum as foreign bodies are unable to pass through the physiological angulation [20].

Although emergent surgical intervention is often the first line treatment for perforation, there are case reports in the literature that discuss endoscopic management [18]. Simunic et al. discussed the successful endoscopic retrieval of a sharp foreign body from the cecum that caused a localized perforation [18]. Their report emphasizes that clinically stable patients with localized findings on CT scan are more likely to be successfully managed using this technique. Despite case reports discussing the management of localized perforations, foreign body ingestions that present as perforations do not usually manifest with minimal symptoms and clinical stability. Consideration of endoscopic management should be on a case by case basis if the appropriate qualified personnel are available to assist in treatment. Overall, surgical treatment is still the recommended course of treatment for such complications.

4.2 Obstruction

The literature regarding foreign body ingestion causing obstruction is relatively limited to case series at single institutions and published case reports. Review of the available literature supports that intestinal perforation is the most common presenting complication with obstruction being the second most frequently encountered [21].

As mentioned previously, delayed presentation following foreign body ingestion increases the risks for complications, such as intestinal obstruction. In patients who present in a delayed fashion after ingestion of superabsorbent polymers, as the time increases following ingestion, both the length of passage and amount of water absorbed by the foreign body increases. These factors increase the likelihood of intestinal obstruction and decrease the chance that the foreign body will pass without either endoscopic or surgical intervention [2]. The key to preventing intestinal obstruction is to pursue endoscopic intervention early when ingestion is highly suspected but not witnessed. If obstruction is not identified in a timely fashion, then it can lead to intestinal perforation, which has its own associated morbidity.

4.3 Bleeding

Most complications reported in the literature associated with foreign body ingestion are related to perforation, obstruction, or fistula formation. Bleeding is another complication that can result from foreign body ingestion. Hemorrhage can result from direct mucosal injury from sharp objects. Bleeding may also occur due to erosion of the mucosa caused by blunt objects. In patients who are hemodynamically stable and present with gastrointestinal bleeding with a history of foreign body ingestion, endoscopic intervention should be considered not only as a diagnostic tool but also as potentially therapeutic.

The ESGE recommends that endoscopy be performed within 24 hours for sharp and long objects that are in the stomach to prevent complications such as bleeding, perforation, and obstruction. In the pediatric population it is well documented that button batteries, if ingested, may lead to all the above complications [1]. Although, they are most commonly lodged in the esophagus, if they do pass into the stomach and then into the small intestine, they may cause obstruction leading to mucosal erosion and subsequently perforation. A patient may present with hematemesis or lower GI bleed depending on where the object is causing mucosal erosion. It is estimated that the risk of complications can be as high as 35% once these objects leave the stomach [1]. With regards to adult literature, case reports have been published showing that ingestion of sharp foreign bodies can cause life-threatening gastrointestinal bleeding. Gattai et al. reported on a patient who had ingested glass, which caused lacerations in the fourth portion of the duodenum that led to a severe gastrointestinal bleed. During operative intervention the patient was found to have a segment of jejunal diverticulum; however, the source of bleeding was not found in the resected portion of bowel. Following small bowel resection, the patient continued to hemorrhage and was found to have active bleeding from lacerations found in the duodenum. This case report demonstrates the severity of foreign body ingestion and appropriate surgical management [22]. If bleeding is unable to be controlled endoscopically, then surgical intervention is mandated. Although gastrointestinal hemorrhage is a rare complication, its morbidity should not be underestimated.

5. Special considerations

Bezoars are uncommon masses formed from indigestible ingested substances in the gastrointestinal system. They were named in 1854 by Quain, after a mass of intragastric food residue was found during autopsy [23]. They are reported to contribute to up to 4% of small bowel obstructions [23–25]. Many are diagnosed post-operatively as they do not have a clinically significant difference in presentation from other causes of small bowel obstruction [24]. There are different forms of bezoars that are classified based on the content that forms the mass.

5.1 Classification

There are five types of bezoars: phytobezoars, trichobezoars, polybezoars, pharmacobezoars, and lactobezoars [23, 25]. Phytobezoars are made of vegetable and fruit residues, trichobezoars consist of hair, a lactobezoar is formed from dairy products, polybezoars are caused by ingested foreign bodies, and a pharmacobezoar is caused by medications [23]. The most common type of bezoar is the phytobezoar, which typically consists of cellulose and hemicellulose from indigestible food residue [23]. Trichobezoars are generally seen in individuals with trichophagia, a psychiatric disorder that causes the compulsive eating of hair after pulling (trichotillomania), usually seen in young adults and during childhood [23, 26, 27]. Most cases of trichobezoars are reported in females, which may be attributed to the tendency to have longer hair [26]. These bezoars are generally located in the stomach, but prolonged or unrecognized ingestion can cause a process known as Rapunzel syndrome, where the hair extends from the stomach into the small intestine [23, 26, 27]. Treatment of the underlying psychiatric illness is paramount to prevent recurrence and further complication. Trichobezoar with Rapunzel syndrome is an uncommon diagnosis in children, with fewer than 100 cases reported [26].

5.2 Presentation

The symptoms of bezoars can differ according to size, location and the level of obstruction. Gastric bezoars will usually present with vomiting, upper abdominal pain and distention, which are common symptoms of obstruction [23, 24]. The most common symptom has been reported as upper abdominal pain [24]. It is often difficult to differentiate small bowel obstruction (SBO) secondary to bezoar from adhesive obstruction in a patient who has had previous abdominal surgery.

The history portion of the clinical exam is often the most important in this patient population as past surgical history and medical conditions can raise suspicion for a bezoar. Predisposing factors of bowel obstruction due to bezoar are ingestion of a high-fiber diet, abnormal chewing, diminished gastric secretion and motility, diabetics, patients with myotonic dystrophy and many other less common factors [23–25]. High-fiber foods such as celery, pumpkins, grape skins, prunes and especially persimmons, are a risk factor for formation [23]. Bezoars are prevalent among patients with delayed gastric emptying such as after a gastrectomy or a vagotomy, or secondary to diabetic autonomic neuropathy and hypothyroidism [23–25]. Bezoar causing SBO in patients with previous gastric surgery is well known as a late complication, although rare [25]. Incidence of post-gastrectomy bezoar has been reported to be between 5 and 15%, and the time it takes a bezoar to form after gastric surgery ranges from 9 months to 30 years [23, 25]. Bezoars can also be formed primarily in the small intestine when a mechanical factor alters the small intestinal lumen such as a diverticulum, tumor or stricture [23]. Pharmacobezoars are usually caused by Kayexalate (sodium polystyrene sulfonate), cholestyramine and antacid medications [23]. Lactobezoars typically occur in low-birth-weight newborns as a result of concentrated baby formulas [23].

An accurate preoperative diagnosis is often difficult due to lack of specific symptoms, and clinical presentation of an acute surgical abdomen is very rare, occurring in 1.1% of cases [24, 25]. Most bezoars in the small bowel are found approximately 50 to 70 cm above the ileocecal valve because of narrowing with slower intestinal motility and significant water absorption that hardens the bezoar [24]. The most common site of obstruction is the terminal ileum [25].

5.3 Imaging

Computed-tomography is the gold standard imaging modality for diagnosing small bowel obstruction due to bezoar [23, 24]. Contrast-enhanced CT imaging is the most valuable method for determining the location and etiology of intestinal obstructions [23]. The history provided by the patient in conjunction with CT imaging findings will likely give the most complete picture. As many bezoars can be radiolucent, plain film radiographs may have less utility. Other imaging modalities that can be considered are abdominal ultrasound, which has a reportedly high diagnostic rate of 88–93%, but this is user dependent and can be limited by patient's body habitus, gas accumulation and location of the obstruction [24].

5.4 Treatment

Treatment is identical to that previously described for other forms of small bowel obstruction due to foreign body ingestion. The minimally invasive approach of endoscopy, including double-balloon enteroscopy, may be used as a first line if the patient is stable without perforation. Case reports have described the use of endoscopic fragmentation, gastric lavage, enzymatic therapy or combination of these approaches [26, 27]. Bezoars like Rapunzel syndrome require surgical removal. Laparoscopic enterotomy and retrieval should be considered for any obstructions not amenable to endoscopic treatment. Open surgical management should be reserved for patients in extremis, with perforation and contamination, or based on the availability of experienced endoscopic and laparoscopic surgeons and resources.

6. Conclusions

Foreign body ingestion can be a challenge to manage. It creates diagnostic as well as treatment dilemmas for clinicians. Evaluation should be initiated with a basic history and physical exam, and further imaging studies should be obtained based on the information gathered. After appropriate work-up has been completed, clinicians can determine the next step in management. Most foreign body ingestions may be managed non-operatively; however, in some situations, management may be a multidisciplinary approach that includes gastroenterologists and surgeons. Ultimately, the patient's clinical stability and examination should determine the best course in management to prevent complications associated with foreign body ingestion.

Acknowledgements

We would like to express our thanks to Dr Brian Daley for his guidance. We appreciate his patience and time. We would also like to thank the University of

Tennessee Graduate School of Medicine for providing us with the resources to compile the research used in the content of this manuscript. No source of funding was used in the production of this manuscript.

Conflict of interest

The authors declare no conflict of interest.

Author details

Jessica Elizabeth Taylor* and Devin Clegg
University of Tennessee Graduate School of Medicine, Knoxville, TN, United States

*Address all correspondence to: jtaylor4@utmck.edu

References

[1] Birk M, Bauerfeind P, Deprez PH, et al. Removal of foreign bodies in the upper gastrointestinal tract in adults: European Society of Gastrointestinal Endoscopy (ESGE) clinical guideline. Endoscopy. 2016;**48**:489-496. DOI: 10.1055/s-0042-100456

[2] Kramer RE, Lerner DG, Lin T, et al. Management of ingested foreign bodies in children: A clinical report of the NASPGHAN endoscopy committee. Journal of Pediatric Gastroenterology and Nutrition. 2015;**60**:562-574. DOI: 10.1097/MPG.0000000000000729

[3] Ikenberry SO, Jue TL, Anderson MA, et al. Management of ingested foreign bodies and food impactions. Gastrointestinal Endoscopy. June 2011;**73**:1085-1091. DOI: 10.1016/j.gie.2010.11.010

[4] Arshad M, Jeelani SM, Salim A, et al. Multiple magnet ingestion leading to bowel perforation: A relatively sinister foreign body. Cureus. 2019;**11**:e5866. DOI: 10.7759/cureus.5866

[5] Kozaci N, Avci M, Pinarbasili T, et al. Ingested foreign body imaging using point-of-care ultrasonography: A case series. Pediatric Emergency Care. 2019;**35**:807-810. DOI: 10.1097/PEC.0000000000001971

[6] Taylor JE, Campbell M, Daley B. The management of small bowel obstruction caused by ingested gastrostomy tube. The American Surgeon. 2019;**85**(8):e372-e373

[7] Eisen GM, Baron TH, Dominitz JA, et al. Guideline for the management of ingested foreign bodies. Gastrointestinal Endoscopy. 2002;**55**(7):802-806. DOI: 10.1016/s0016-5107(02)70407-0

[8] Mulholland MW, Lillemoe KD, Doherty GM, Upchurch GR Jr, Alam HB, Pawlik TM, editors. Other childhood gastrointestinal disorders. In: Greenfield's Surgery: Scientific Principles & Practice. 6th ed. Philadelphia: Lippincott Williams & Wilkins; 2016. p. 1904-1914

[9] Wnęk B, Łożyńska-Nelke A, Karoń J. Foreign body in the gastrointestinal tract leading to small bowel obstruction—Case report and literature review. Polish Journal of Surgery. 2015;**86**(12):549-597. DOI: 10.1515/pjs-2015-0006

[10] Yao C-C, Wu I-T, Lu L-S, et al. endoscopic management of foreign bodies in the upper gastrointestinal tract of adults. BioMed Research International. 2015;**2015**:1-6. DOI: 10.1155/2015/658602

[11] Di Saverio S, Bianchini Massoni C, Boschi S, et al. Complete small-bowel obstruction from a migrated intra-gastric balloon: Emergency laparoscopy for retrieval via enterotomy and intra-corporeal repair. Obesity Surgery. 2014;**24**(10):1830-1832. DOI: 10.1007/s11695-014-1271-5

[12] Nakamura M, Hirooka Y, Watanabe O, et al. Minimally invasive extraction of a foreign body from the small intestine using double-balloon endoscopy. Nagoya Journal of Medical Science. 2015;**77**(1-2):189-194

[13] Kay M, Wyllie R. Foreign body ingestions in the pediatric population and techniques of endoscopic removal. Techniques in Gastrointestinal Endoscopy. 2013;**15**(1):9-17. DOI: 10.1016/j.tgie.2012.09.005

[14] Chia DKA, Wijaya R, Wong A, Tan S-M. Laparoscopic management of complicated foreign body ingestion: A case series. International Surgery. 2015;**100**(5):849-853. DOI: 10.9738/INTSURG-D-14-00238.1

[15] Mohamed Aboulkacem B, Ghalleb M, Khemir A, et al. Laparoscopic assisted foreign body

extraction from the small bowel: A case report. International Journal of Surgery Case Reports. 2017;**41**:283-286. DOI: 10.1016/j.ijscr.2017.08.047

[16] Mulholland MW, Lillemoe KD, Doherty GM, Upchurch GR Jr, Alam HB, Pawlik TM, editors. Mechanical obstruction of the intestines. In: Greenfield's Surgery: Scientific Principles & Practice. 6th ed. pp. 782-798

[17] Alsharief AN, Blackmore C, Schmit P. Small bowel obstruction due to ingestion of rubber balls. Pediatric Radiology. 2017;**47**(11):1539-1541. DOI: 10.1007/s00247-017-3894-x

[18] Simunic M, Zaja I, Ardalic Z, et al. Case report: Successful endoscopic treatment of a large bowel perforation caused by chicken bone ingestion. Medicine. 2019;**98**:e18111. DOI: 10.1097/MD.0000000000018111

[19] Rodríguez-Hermosa JI, Codina-Cazador A, Sirvent JM, et al. Surgically treated perforations of the gastrointestinal tract caused by ingested foreign bodies. Colorectal Disease. 2008;**10**:701-707

[20] Li C, Yong CC, Encarnacion DD. Duodenal perforation nine months after accidental foreign body ingestion, a case report. BMC Surgery. 2019;**19**:132. DOI: 10.1186/s12893-019-0594-5

[21] Shao F, Shen N, Hong Z, et al. Injuries due to foreign body ingestion and insertion in children: 10 years of experience at a single institution. Journal of Paediatrics and Child Health. 2019;**56**:537-541. DOI: 10.1111/jpc.14677

[22] Gattai R, Pantalone D, Migliaccio ML, Bonizzoli M, Peris A, Bechi P. Upper G.I. hemorrhage from glass fragments' ingestion in a patient with jejunal diverticula—Case report. International Journal of Surgery Case Reports. 2015;**6C**:191-193. DOI: 10.1016/j.ijscr.2014.11.069

[23] Dikicier E. Intestinal obstruction due to phytobezoars: An update. World Journal of Clinical Cases. 2015;**3**(8):721. DOI: 10.12998/wjcc.v3.i8.721

[24] Oh SH, Namgung H, Park MH, Park D-G. Bezoar-induced small bowel obstruction. Journal of the Korean Society of Coloproctology. 2012;**28**(2):89. DOI: 10.3393/jksc.2012.28.2.89

[25] Nasri B, Calin M, Shah A, Gilchrist B. A rare cause of small bowel obstruction due to bezoar in a virgin abdomen. International Journal of Surgery Case Reports. 2016;**19**:144-146. DOI: 10.1016/j.ijscr.2015.12.039

[26] Gonuguntla V, Joshi D-D. Rapunzel syndrome: A comprehensive review of an unusual case of trichobezoar. Clinical Medicine & Research. 2009;**7**(3):99-102. DOI: 10.3121/cmr.2009.822

[27] Al-Janabi IS, Al-Sharbaty MA, Al-Sharbati MM, Al-Sharifi LA, Ouhtit A. Unusual trichobezoar of the stomach and the intestine: A case report. Journal of Medical Case Reports. 2014;**8**(1):79. DOI: 10.1186/1752-1947-8-79

Chapter 5

Caecal Volvulus

Paul K. Okeny

Abstract

Colonic volvulus is the third leading cause of large bowel obstruction. About 35% of these are located in the caecum. Though, relatively, a rare cause of obstruction, the incidence of caecal volvulus is steadily increasing at a rate of about 5% per year. Mortality due to caecal volvulus may be as high as 40% especially in the presence of gangrene and sepsis. Clinical presentation may be acute and fulminant or as a mobile caecum syndrome with intermittent abdominal pain. "Whirl," "Coffee bean," and "bird beak" signs seen on computed tomography are pathognomonic. Colectomy is the preferred treatment as it obviates any chance of recurrence. A conservative approach to colectomy such as limited ileocaecal resection and ileostomy formation in critically ill patients or in those with poor physiological reserve may be associated with better postoperative outcomes.

Keywords: caecum, volvulus, obstruction, mobile caecum, management

1. Introduction

There are records of volvulus as far back as 1550 BC and by Hippocrates who first described treatment options such as injection of a large quantity of air or insertion of a 10 digit suppository through the anus [1]. In modern day literature, it was first described by Austrian pathologist Rokitansky in 1837 as an important cause of intestinal strangulation [2]. Colonic volvulus or twisting of the large bowel is the third leading cause of large bowel obstruction world-wide [3]. It mainly occurs in the 'Volvulus belt' of Africa, Middle East, India and Russia where it may affect a slightly younger age group compared to the rest of the world [4, 5].

Although the incidence of caecal volvulus as a cause of colonic volvulus appears to be increasing, the commonest sites for colonic volvulus still include sigmoid –60%, caecum –35%, transverse colon –4%, and splenic flexure –1% [1]. This chapter reviews the current management of caecal volvulus.

2. Epidemiology

Caecal volvulus in itself is rare but an associated mortality of nearly 40% warrants prompt diagnosis and treatment [6]. It has an incidence of 2.8–7.1 per million people, is responsible for 1–1.5% of intestinal obstructions, and 25–40% of all colonic volvulus and affects females more than males [7]. The presence of a volvulus belt has already been discussed. In a large epidemiological study done by Halabi et al. [8] over a period covering 9 years in the United States, the incidence of caecal volvulus increased by 5% per year.

3. Aetiology

The aetiology of caecal volvulus can be attributed to an interplay between anatomical and other predisposing factors.

In normal embryological development, the mesentery of the right colon gets fixed on the right posterior abdominal wall (retroperitoneum) during the counter clockwise rotation of the caecum from left to right lower quadrant. Abnormal fixation may lead to an excessively mobile caecum in an anatomical anomaly called “messenterium commune” [9]. In an autopsy examination of 125 cadavers, 11.2% had freely mobile colons with a 36.8% total risk of caecal volvulus [3, 10].

Including previous surgery – adhesions acting as fulcrum for rotation of the mobile caecum [11], other predisposing factors include chronic constipation, distal obstruction, prior colonoscopy, high fibre diet, psychotropic drugs, ileus and late term pregnancy [7, 10, 12–14].

The commonest features in the aetiology of caecal volvulus are therefore caecal displacement, hyperperistalsis/dysmotility and colonic distension. It may also be associated with other congenital malformations such as Cornelia de Lange in children [15] and situs inversus [16].

4. Pathophysiology

Caecal volvulus occurs when the caecum which forms the first part of the large bowel undergoes an axial twist about its mesenteric pedicle leading to a closed loop intestinal obstruction [7, 17]. Also involved in this process are the ascending colon and terminal ileum. This should be differentiated from caecal bascule in which the caecum folds anteriorly along a horizontal plane [7, 18, 19]. See **Figures 1–3**.

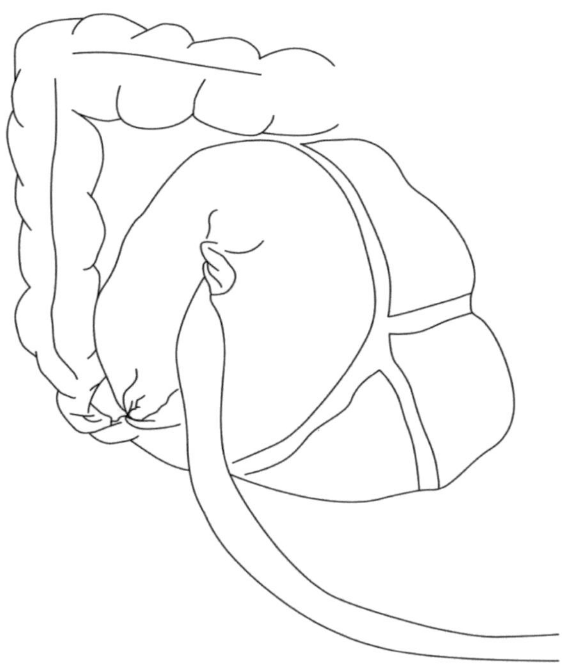

Figure 1.
Caecal volvulus with axial twist causing closed loop obstruction. Adapted from Consorti and Liu [7].

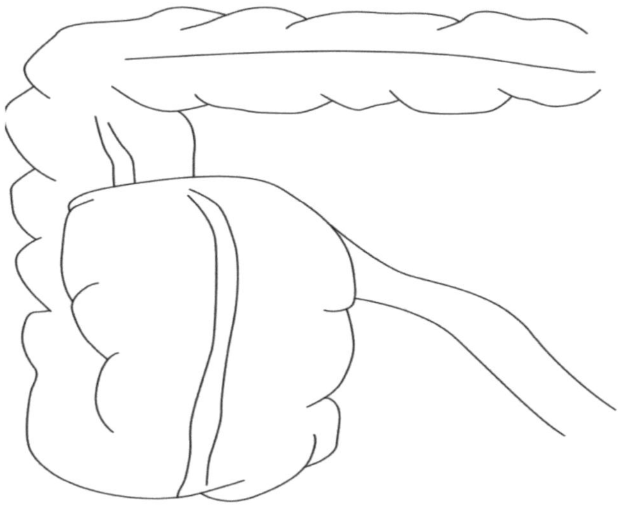

Figure 2.
Caecal bascule. Upward fold along horizontal plane. Adapted from Consorti and Liu [7].

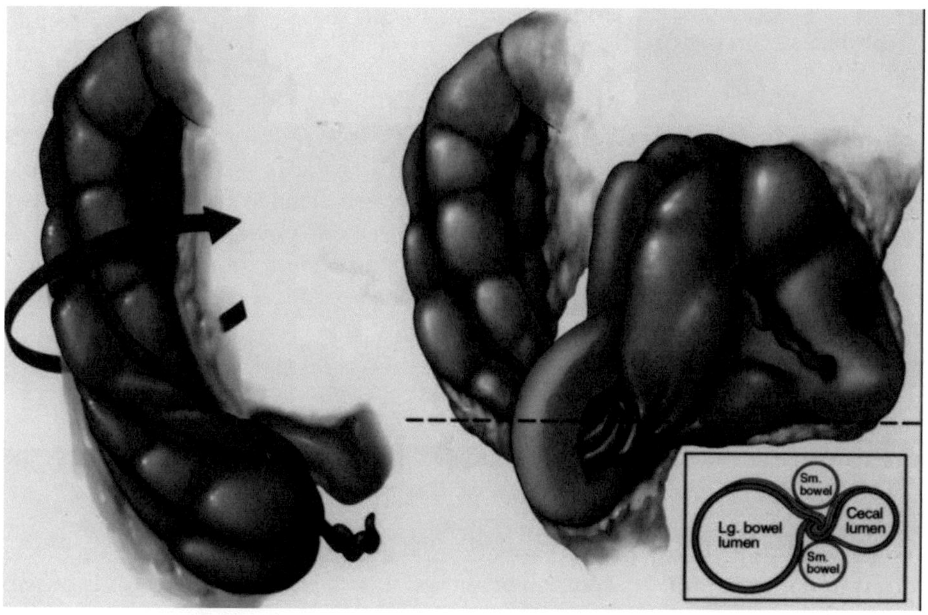

Figure 3.
Pictorial illustration of loop type caecal volvulus with entangled terminal ileum from Moore et al. [22] inset illustrates 'whirl sign' at the point of obstruction/torsion as seen in CT images.

Many scholars report three types of caecal volvulus [20–22]:

- Type 1 in which a clockwise axial twist results in the volvulus being located in the right lower quadrant.
- Type 2 in which both the caecum and terminal ileum get involved and ectopically located in the Left upper quadrant in an inverted position. Here, the caecum both twists and inverts and this twist may sometimes be counter clockwise [22]. This type is also referred to as the 'loop type' of caecal volvulus. It results in a characteristically empty right iliac fossa [23].

- Type 3 caecal volvulus also known as caecal bascule, is characterised by absence of axial twist.

In all these types, there is potential for intestinal obstruction and strangulation [11, 24] with the risk higher in types 1 and 2 which constitute about 80% of caecal volvulus. Caecal volvulus may sometimes coexist with a synchronous splenic flexure volvulus [25] and/or sigmoid volvulus [26].

Baumann et al. [27] propose a mathematical model based on the physics of a spring to explain the mechanism of occurrence of exercise related caecal volvulus in long distance runners and aggressive walkers. Repetitive vertical stretching of caecum and ascending colon leads to loss of elastic recoil and a laxed mesentery which predisposes to volvulus.

5. Clinical presentation

The clinical presentation of caecal volvulus can be divided into separate but interrelated clinical syndromes that is, mobile caecum syndrome, acute obstruction and acute fulminant obstruction [7].

5.1 Mobile caecum syndrome

This may be associated with caecal bascule and occurs due to increased mobility of the caecum. It is characterised by recurrent, intermittent abdominal pain and distension which typically resolves on passage of flatus [18, 28]. Vomiting may occur in only 30% of the patients [18]. It may be associated with some functional colon diseases such as chronic constipation and irritable bowel syndrome.

Gomes et al. [29] propose a laparoscopic grading system for mobile caecum syndrome depending on the degree of mobility of the ileocaecal and appendiceal unit:

- Grade I – The peritoneal attachments are intact and the unit is within the right iliac fossa and does not cross the midline.

- Grade II – The ileocaecal and appendiceal unit can easily be moved across the midline. No fixation hence axial twist about its own axis is possible.

- Grade III – The ileocaecal and appendiceal unit can easily be moved up to the left upper quadrant. No fixation hence axial twist about its own axis is possible.

Caecopexy is advised for Grades II and III.

Due to the quick resolution of symptoms, diagnosis of the mobile cecum syndrome can be difficult. Cesaretti et al. [28] advise performing computed tomography in Trendelenburg position and propose use of virtual colonoscopy to aid diagnosis of mobile caecum syndrome.

Up to 50% of patients with acute obstructive caecal volvulus tend to initially present with features of mobile caecum syndrome [30, 31].

5.2 Acute obstructive pattern

This may be simple – no ischaemia, or fulminant obstruction – bowel ischaemia, sepsis and peritonitis.

These patients present with classical features of acute intestinal obstruction that is, abdominal pain, distension, constipation and vomiting. Being the first part of large bowel clinical features of caecal volvulus may be indistinguishable from those of acute small bowel obstruction.

In simple obstruction, patients may present with dehydration and electrolyte imbalance due to persistent vomiting. Prolonged obstruction may result in strangulation, gangrene and perforation. At this point patients are toxic, peritonitic, septic and in metabolic acidosis.

The sepsis is associated with translocation of bacteria due to a damaged caecal/colonic mucosal layer. This damage is due to mechanical cut off of arterial blood supply or severe caecal distension –>10 cm with intraluminal pressure greatly exceeding mucosal capillary pressure.

Nearly 30% of the acute obstructive pattern occurs in hospitalised patients [32, 33]. This may be attributed to bowel distension and dysmotility. Symptoms in these patients may be masked by the signs and symptoms of concurrent medical illness. High index of suspicion and early diagnostic imaging are therefore paramount [7].

6. Evaluation

Following a thorough history and physical examination, a laboratory workup and appropriate diagnostic imaging should be planned while resuscitation is on-going. The surgeon should be sure to take medication history and ascertain pre-existing comorbidities to ensure they are under control. It is important at this point to pass a urethral catheter and monitor fluid input/output, pass a nasogastric tube if there is excessive distension with vomiting and administer antiemetics and analgesics.

7. Laboratory workup

These are usually non-specific. However, a complete blood count (CBC) with differential, metabolic panel, lactic acid, urea and electrolytes should be done. Fluid and electrolyte imbalance may be found in patients who have had prolonged obstruction with vomiting, bowel ischaemia, peritonitis or systemic sepsis.

8. Radiology

8.1 Plain abdominal radiography (AXR)

In many limited resource settings, this may be the only available radiological investigation. However, the plain AXR is diagnostic in less than 20% of the cases [11, 34] and sometimes the surgeon's only option is to perform an emergency exploratory celiotomy. In cases where AXR is diagnostic or suggestive of caecal volvulus, the typical findings include caecal distension in over 98%, absence of gas in distal colon in 82%, a distended small bowel in 55% that is pushed lateral to the caecum and a single air-fluid level in the right lower quadrant [11]. In contrast to sigmoid volvulus, haustrations are nearly always visible in caecal volvulus. James and Kelly [35] provide an extensive account on how to perform and interpret abdominal radiographs.

8.2 Barium Enema (BE)

This was traditionally used for diagnosis and treatment of colonic volvulus including caecal volvulus [11]. It had the advantage of being 88% accurate and the possibility of visualising the distal colon for any obstructive causes of volvulus. The "bird beak sign" in the efferent limb is diagnostic [36]. However, it has now been abandoned due to time needed to perform and potential for extravasation of contrast. Currently, a water soluble contrast such as gastrograffin enema may be used [37]. It is absolutely contraindicated in critically ill patients and in suspected perforation or strangulation.

8.3 Computed tomography (CT) scan

Abdominopelvic CT scan is currently the imaging of choice for diagnosis of caecal volvulus. Rosenblatt et al. [38] and later Dane et al. [39] provide an extensive discussion on the utility of CT findings in the diagnosis of caecal volvulus. The CT findings more common in caecal volvulus included severe caecal distension ≥10 cm, whirl sign, abnormal caecal position, central appendix – at or close to the midline, split wall, coffee bean sign and distal colonic decompression. In the study conducted by Dane et al., [39] the whirl sign was an independent predictor of caecal volvulus. The "whirl," "coffee bean" and "bird beak" signs are considered pathognomonic for caecal volvulus although a gas filled appendix is also a common finding especially in the loop type of caecal volvulus [22]. Findings of pneumatosis intestinalis and portal venous gas are suggestive of bowel ischaemia.

8.4 Colonoscopy

In contrast to sigmoid volvulus, the role of colonoscopy in diagnosis and treatment of caecal volvulus is very limited and has a reported success rate of less than 30%. It is associated with delay in definitive operative treatment and high risk for perforation hence not generally recommended [24, 40].

Despite all the above investigations and the high sensitivity and specificity of CT scan for diagnosis of caecal volvulus, diagnosis can sometimes only be made intraoperatively in about 10% of the cases [24, 39, 41].

9. Treatment

Definitive treatment should be sought as soon as the patient has been adequately resuscitated. The surgeon has to decide between non-operative and operative treatment.

9.1 Non-operative treatment

Absolute contraindications to non-operative treatment include pneumoperitoneum, bowel ischaemia, peritonitis or clinically confirmed tenderness over the distended caecum. In very elderly, frail patients with multiple comorbidities and advanced obstruction, the risks of an operation may outweigh the benefits. In such situations, the surgical team may decide to offer palliation. This decision must be reached after consideration of availability of resources for peri and postoperative care and in conjunction with the patient and/or family.

As stated earlier, the role of colonoscopy is generally limited and more than 90% of patients will require surgical treatment. There have been a few reports of successful detorsion of caecal volvulus especially in children albeit with recurrence as early as 6 weeks after colonoscopy [42, 43].

Barium enema is currently not recommended for treatment of caecal volvulus.

9.2 Operative treatment

The surgical approach may be open – midline laparotomy, or laparoscopic depending on availability of resources, surgeon's expertise and patient factors.

A laparoscopic approach is currently considered safe in both the acute and elective setting [28, 37]. In a series of 15 patients with mobile caecum syndrome who underwent laparoscopic caecopexy, Gomes et al. [29] report a very favourable outcome with 84% achieving a modified Visick score [44] of 1 while up to 92% had only a Grade I Clavien-Dindo classification [45].

Most of the time, an emergency laparotomy may be needed especially in fulminant cases even precluding diagnostic imaging. In all cases, an honest discussion needs to be held preoperatively with the patient and their family regarding possible outcomes given available resources. The surgical team will need to be proactive and invite the intensive care team (ICU) for peri and postoperative care planning as some of these patients may require postoperative care in the ICU.

At laparotomy, the decision regarding definitive treatment relies heavily on the operating surgeon and their experience [7]. The factors affecting these decisions are mainly the patient's physiological reserve and state of the bowel. The surgical options are:

- Detorsion and/or caecopexy
- Caecostomy – decompresses caecum and fixes it on to the anterior abdominal wall.
- Resection and primary anastomosis – this may be the traditional right hemicolectomy or a more limited ileocaecal resection with or without colopexy of the right colon.
- Resection and temporary ileostomy or ileostomy with mucus fistula.

There are no randomized controlled trials comparing these treatment options. However, in the presence of gangrene – which occurs about 23 to nearly 100% of the time [24], overly distended and stretched caecum, resection is mandatory. It is advisable not to untwist the gangrenous portion in order not to release toxins into the blood circulation that would lead to worsening of septic shock [46].

Overall mortality with resectional procedures is up to 32% [24]. In patients with poor physiological reserve, a conservative approach such as limited ileocaecal resection or formation of an ileostomy may reduce intraoperative time and result in better postoperative outcome [47]. In synchronous caecal and sigmoid volvulus, a total colectomy with ileostomy may sometimes be necessary [26].

Detorsion alone is associated with a recurrence of up to 75% [24]. A combination of detorsion and caecopexy greatly reduces this recurrence rate to less than 15% with a mortality of about 10% [11]. The technique of caecopexy involves placing two to three knots to attach the lateral taenia coli of the caecum or right colon in colopexy to the right paracolic gutter approximately along the level of the axillary line [29]. This may be achieved by initially raising a peritoneal flap at this level as in the Dixon and Meyer's approach [48]. Sakamoto et al. [49] report a successful case of percutaneous endoscopic colopexy in caecal volvulus.

Caecostomy alone is associated with a mortality of 22% and a recurrence rate of 14–20% [11]. It is advised as a temporary measure or in very high-risk surgical candidates. The technique involves catheter or tube decompression of the caecum through the anterior abdominal wall. The catheters may regularly get blocked due to the viscid faeces and may require regular flushing. Alternatively, a wider more rigid size 8–9 mm endotracheal tube may be ballooned, sutured in place and attached to an ordinary urinary bag [50]. The approach to caecostomy may be percutaneous – endoscopic or needle [51, 52], or during formal laparotomy.

10. Conclusion

Caecal volvulus is a rare but important cause of intestinal obstruction. It is both organ and life threatening especially if advanced and fulminant. Abdominopelvic CT scan is the preferred imaging and the "whirl sign" is an independent predictor of caecal volvulus. The choice of surgical option hugely depends on the operating surgeon. Current advances favour a multidisciplinary approach and colectomy as the choice of treatment following adequate resuscitation. The surgeon should work closely with the intensive care team as some of these patients may require postoperative mechanical ventilation. Both patient and/or family preferences need to be considered during the course of management.

Conflict of interest

None.

Author details

Paul K. Okeny
School of Postgraduate Studies, Royal College of Surgeons in Ireland, Dublin, Ireland

*Address all correspondence to: PaulOkeny@rcsi.ie; okenykpaul@yahoo.ca

References

[1] Ballantyne GH. Review of sigmoid volvulus: History and results of treatment. Diseases of the Colon and Rectum. 1982;**25**(5):494-501

[2] Rokitansky C. Intestinal strangulation. Archives of General Internal Medicine. 1837;**14**:202-204

[3] Ballantyne GH, Brandner MD, Beart RW Jr, Ilstrup DM. Volvulus of the colon. Incidence and mortality. Annals of Surgery. 1985;**202**(1):83-92

[4] Heis HA, Bani-Hani KE, Rabadi DK, Elheis MA, Bani-Hani BK, Mazahreh TS, et al. Sigmoid volvulus in the Middle East. World Journal of Surgery. 2008;**32**(3):459-464

[5] Bruusgaard C. Volvulus of the sigmoid colon and its treatment. Surgery. 1947;**22**(3):466-478

[6] Renzulli P, Maurer CA, Netzer P, Büchler MW. Preoperative colonoscopic derotation is beneficial in acute colonic volvulus. Digestive Surgery. 2002;**19**:223-229

[7] Consorti ET, Liu TH. Diagnosis and treatment of caecal volvulus. Postgraduate Medical Journal. 2005;**81**:772-776

[8] Halabi WJ, Jafari MD, Kang CY, Nguyen VQ, Carmichael JC, Mills S, et al. Colonic volvulus in the United States: Trends, outcomes, and predictors of mortality. Annals of Surgery. 2014;**259**(2):293-301

[9] Moritz AR. Mesenterium commune with intestinal obstruction. The American Journal of Pathology. 1932;**8**(6):735-744.1

[10] Gingold D, Murrell Z. Management of colonic volvulus. Clinics in Colon and Rectal Surgery. 2012;**25**(4):236-244

[11] Rabinovici R, Simansky DA, Kaplan O, Mavor E, Manny J. Cecal volvulus. Diseases of the Colon and Rectum. 1990;**33**(9):765-769

[12] Montes H, Wolf J. Cecal volvulus in pregnancy. The American Journal of Gastroenterology. 1999;**94**:2554-2555

[13] Tejler G, Jiborn H. Volvulus of the cecum. Report of 26 cases and review of the literature. Diseases of the Colon and Rectum. 1988;**31**:445-449

[14] Viney R, Fordan SV, Fisher WE, Ergun G. Cecal volvulus after colonoscopy. The American Journal of Gastroenterology. 2002;**97**(12):3211-3212

[15] Miura da Costa K, Saxena AK. A systematic review of the management and outcomes of cecal and appendiceal volvulus in children. Acta Paediatrica. 2018;**107**(12):2054-2058

[16] Elsharif M, Basu I, Phillips D. A case of triple volvulus. Annals of the Royal College of Surgeons of England. 2012;**94**(2):e62-ee4

[17] Majeski J. Operative therapy for cecal volvulus combining resection with colopexy. American Journal of Surgery. 2005;**189**(2):211-213

[18] Lung BE, Yelika SB, Murthy AS, Gachabayov M, Denoya P. Cecal bascule: A systematic review of the literature. Techniques in Coloproctology. 2018;**22**(2):75-80

[19] Park J-S, Ng K-S, Young CJ. Caecal bascule: A case series and literature review. ANZ Journal of Surgery. 2018;**88**(5):E386-E3E9

[20] Le CK, Qaja E. Caecal Volvulus Treasure Island: StatPearls; 2019 [updated 28 February 2019]

[21] Delabrousse E, Sarlière P, Sailley N, Aubry S, Kastler BA. Cecal volvulus: CT findings and correlation with pathophysiology. Emergency Radiology. 2007;**14**(6):411-415

[22] Moore CJ, Corl FM, Fishman EK. CT of cecal volvulus. American Journal of Roentgenology. 2001;**177**(1):95-98

[23] Zabeirou AA, Belghali H, Souiki T, Ibn Majdoub K, Toughrai I, Mazaz K. Acute cecal volvulus: A diagnostic and therapeutic challenge in emergency: A case report. Annals of Medicine and Surgery. 2019;**48**:69-72

[24] Madiba TE, Thomson SR. The management of cecal volvulus. Diseases of the Colon and Rectum. 2002;**45**(2):264-267

[25] Islam S, Hosein D, Harnarayan P, Naraynsingh V. Synchronic volvulus of splenic flexure and caecum: A very rare cause of large bowel obstruction. BMJ Case Reports. 2016;**2016**:bcr2015-213029

[26] Roy SP, Tay YK, Kozman D. Very rare case of synchronous volvulus of the sigmoid colon and caecum causing large-bowel obstruction. BML Case Reports. 2019;**12**(1):bcr-2018-227375

[27] Bauman BD, Witt JE, Vakayil V, Anwer S, Irwin ED, Kwaan MR, et al. Cecal volvulus in long-distance runners: A proposed mechanism. The American Journal of Emergency Medicine. 2019;**37**(3):549-552

[28] Cesaretti M, Trotta M, Leale I, Minetti GA, Cittadini G, Montecucco F, et al. Surgery to treat symptomatic mobile cecum syndrome is safe and associated with good recovery outcomes. Case Reports in Gastrointestinal Medicine. 2018;**2018**:4718406

[29] Gomes CA, Soares C Jr, Catena F, Di Saverio S, Sartelli M, Gomes CC, et al. Laparoscopic Management of Mobile Cecum. JSLS. 2016;**20**(4):e2016.00076

[30] Rogers RL, Harford FJ. Mobile cecum syndrome. Diseases of the Colon and Rectum. 1984;**27**(6):399-402

[31] Printen KJ. Mobile cecal syndrome in the adult. The American Surgeon. 1976;**42**(3):204-205

[32] Theuer C, Cheadle WG. Volvulus of the colon. The American Surgeon. 1991;**57**(3):145-150

[33] Friedman JD, Odland MD, Bubrick MP. Experience with colonic volvulus. Diseases of the Colon and Rectum. 1989;**32**(5):409-416

[34] Rakinic J. Colonic volvulus. In: Beck DE, Roberts PL, Saclarides TJ, Senagore AJ, Stamos MJ, Wexner SD, editors. The ASCRS Textbook of Colon and Rectal Surgery. New York, NY: Springer; 2011. pp. 395-406

[35] James B, Kelly B. The abdominal radiograph. The Ulster Medical Journal. 2013;**82**(3):179-187

[36] Young WS. Further radiological observations in caecal volvulus. Clinical Radiology. 1980;**31**(4):479-483

[37] Kelly MD, Bunni J, Pullyblank AM. Laparoscopic assisted right hemicolectomy for caecal volvulus. World Journal of Emergency Surgery. 2008;**3**(1):4

[38] Rosenblat JM, Rozenblit AM, Wolf EL, DuBrow RA, Den EI, Levsky JM. Findings of cecal volvulus at CT. Radiology. 2010;**256**(1):169-175

[39] Dane B, Hindman N, Johnson E, Rosenkrantz AB. Utility of CT findings in the diagnosis of cecal volvulus. American Journal of Roentgenology. 2017;**209**(4):762-766

[40] Anderson MJ, Okike N, Spencer RJ. The colonoscope in cecal volvulus: Report of three cases. Diseases of the Colon and Rectum. 1978;**21**(1):71-74

[41] Pulvirenti E, Palmieri L, Toro A, Carlo ID. Is laparotomy the unavoidable step to diagnose caecal volvulus? Annals of the Royal College of Surgeons of England. 2010;**92**:e27-e29

[42] van de Lagemaat M, Blink M, Bakx R, de Meij TG. Cecal volvulus in children: Is there place for colonoscopic decompression? Journal of Pediatric Gastroenterology and Nutrition. 2018;**66**(2):e59-e60

[43] Shahramian I, Bazil A, Ebadati D, Rostami K, Delaramnasab M. Colonoscopic decompression of childhood sigmoid and cecal volvulus. The Turkish Journal of Gastroenterology. 2018;**29**(2):221-225

[44] Rijnhart-De Jong HG, Draaisma WA, Smout AJ, Broeders IA, Gooszen HG. The Visick score: A good measure for the overall effect of antireflux surgery? Scandinavian Journal of Gastroenterology. 2008;**43**(7):787-793

[45] Dindo D, Demartines N, Clavien PA. Classification of surgical complications: A new proposal with evaluation in a cohort of 6336 patients and results of a survey. Annals of Surgery. 2004;**240**(2):205-213

[46] Tuech JJ, Becouarn G, Cattan F, Arnaud JP. Volvulus of the right colon. Plea for right hemicolectomy. Apropos of a series of 23 cases. J Chir (Paris). 1996;**133**(6):267-269

[47] Kaushal-Deep SM, Anees A, Khan S, Khan MA, Lodhi M. Primary cecal pathologies presenting as acute abdomen and critical appraisal of their current management strategies in emergency settings with review of literature. International Journal of Critical Illness and Injury Science. 2018;**8**(2):90-99

[48] Dixon CF, Meyer AC. Volvulus of the cecum. The Surgical Clinics of North America. 1948;**28**(Mayo Clinic Number):953-963

[49] Sakamoto Y, Hiyoshi Y, Sakata K, Toyama E, Takata N, Yoshinaka I, et al. Case of cecal volvulus successfully treated with endoscopic colopexy. Asian Journal of Endoscopic Surgery. 2018;**11**(4):402-404

[50] Ingoldby CJ, Dawson A, Addison NV. A new technique of caecostomy using endotracheal tubes. Annals of the Royal College of Surgeons of England. 1989;**71**(4):211-212

[51] Koundouris C, Thivaios I, Chrysoulas G, Manisali A, Avitidou E, Sofos G, et al. Percutaneous endoscopic colostomy/caecostomy - A minimally invasive approach to certain colonic disorders: Report of five cases and review of the literature. Hellenic Journal of Surgery. 2016;**88**(2):93-96

[52] Limmer AM, Clement Z. Percutaneous emergency needle Caecostomy for prevention of Caecal perforation. Case Reports in Surgery. 2017;**2017**:1090769

Chapter 6

Sigmoid Volvulus Due Chagas Disease

Víctor Hugo García Orozco

Abstract

American Trypanosomiasis, also known as Chagas disease, is a parasitic disease caused by *Trypanosoma cruzi* and transmitted by hematophagous vectors, occupies the fourth place as a cause of loss of potential years of life between infectious and parasitic diseases, and has an acute presentation form and chronic, in which it can present complications at cardiac and digestive levels, among others. The development of megacolon with subsequent development of volvulus is an important cause of acute abdomen and intestinal obstruction that requires urgent treatment, as it presents an axial rotation of the intestinal loop with obstruction in a closed loop and subsequent ischemia. According to the World Health Organization, there are between 16 and 18 million infected people in the world, of which the majority is located in Latin American territory, and it is estimated that approximately only 1% receives adequate diagnosis and complete treatment.

Keywords: Chagas disease, megacolon, intestinal occlusion, trypanosomiasis, sigmoid volvulus

1. Introduction

Infections and exposure to *Trypanosoma cruzi* occupy the fourth place due to loss of potential years of life between parasitic and infectious diseases [1]. American Trypanosomiasis, also known as Chagas disease, is a parasitic infection transmitted by hematophagous vectors [2] with acute clinical presentation and silent chronic. According to the World Health Organization (WHO), there are between 16 and 18 million infected people in the world, of which the majority is located in Latin American territory, and only 1% receives adequate diagnosis and complete treatment. For the World Health Organization and the Pan American Health Organization, Trypanosomiasis is considered the most serious parasitic disease in Latin America [1].

Transmission can also be done vertically through women infected during pregnancy, which would lead to a congenital disease with intrauterine clinical conditions and at birth.

One of the main complications of the chronic form of Chagas disease is the development of the Chagasic megacolon, which causes alterations in the neurosensory system of the colon. Colon volvulus is described as torsion of the large intestine on its mesenteric axis, thus causing a picture of intestinal obstruction and secondary ischemia.

The development of intestinal volvulations secondary to megacolon [3] is considered as the most severe complication of megacolon syndromes, regardless of

 IntechOpen

their etiology [4]; although it is relatively uncommon in western countries [3], there are records of countries where it occupies the third cause of low intestinal obstruction, only after cancer and diverticular disease [1].

2. Record

Although the vector has been known since the fourteenth century, the first reports of endemia occurred in the post-Columbian period, due to the human displacements that conditioned the direct contact of the vector with the host. In 1909, Dr. Carlos Chagas communicates the discovery of the new human Trypanosomiasis, and in 1911, he obtained the first record of congenital Chagasic disease. In the 1920s, several studies were conducted in pregnant animals that were suffering from acute and chronic stage disease as a follow-up to the theory of vertical transmission [5], and it is in 1949 when Aldao in Venezuela describes the *T. cruzi* finding in peripheral blood of a 2-day-old newborn [2].

The first description with reference to the volvulus was found in the records of Egypt in the Ebers papyrus and mentioned that the volvulus could resolve spontaneously or present a picture of intestinal necrosis; from 1500 BC, it is recognized that detortion of the intestinal loop is crucial for the definitive resolution of the picture, and there are also records made by Hippocrates where suppositories and insufflation were used by mechanical instruments introduced in the anus in order to generate decompression [6]. However, the first description coined with the term Sigmoid volvulus was made by Von Rokitansky in 1836, demonstrating a condition in which the sigmoid wraps itself and its own mesentery, causing a closed loop intestinal obstruction that, if not treated, presented complications such as intestinal ischemia, gangrene, and perforation [7].

Initially, the treatment that was suggested for intestinal torsions was nonsurgical, avoiding intestinal interventions to a greater extent due to the high mortality that occurred in patients with intestinal obstruction; however, after the introduction of aseptic techniques and antisepsis for surgical procedures, in 1883, Atherton performed the first successful surgical procedure for sigmoid volvulus detortion in the United States, and the following year, Treves recommended the colectomy for volvulus that presents vascular complications with gangrene. From 1889, the therapeutic options for volvulus were defined in detortion, pexia, and resection (with or without ostomy) [6].

3. Epidemiological aspects

More than 100 years after the discovery of the causative agent and its form of transmission, Chagas disease is considered the most serious parasitosis in Latin America and one of the 14 lag diseases according to the World Health Organization [8], considering that a minimum of 110 million individuals in 21 countries are at risk of infection. The mother-child transmission of *T. cruzi* can occur at any stage of embryonic and fetal development, without being free of infection none of the periods of development. And although the incidence of vertical transmission in humans is considered low, changes in proportion due to urbanization, migrations from endemic areas and serological controls during transfusions, favor that mother-child transmission is one of the main forms of maintenance of the endemic; however, this form of transmission does not have an exact form of be measured due to nonspecific symptoms and the possibility of going through latent stage for many years. In Argentina, a study was conducted in which it was estimated that, for each case of Vectorial Chagas disease, there would be at least 10 cases of undiagnosed congenital vertical transmission disease [5]. There are estimates that intrauterine infection is considered to be 2–5% of children born to a mother with chronic or latent Chagas disease, while this percentage increases when the infection is acquired during pregnancy and/or when it is associated with immunodeficiency diseases [9]. As mentioned above, there are two fundamental ways of infection, the one caused by vectors and the other that is propitiated vertically from mothers with latent disease, and there are variations regarding the incidence and prevalence rates according to the endemicity of the areas where it presents the disease and population characteristics, as well as the latency and silent disease factor that determines that there may be biases with underestimation or overestimation. Intestinal volvulations are one of the main complications of megacolon (regardless of its etiology), and results in an important cause of intestinal obstruction. Depending on different associated factors such as the height above sea level where patients live, hygienic-dietary habits, racial characteristics, etc., different statistics have been found. A review of the world literature found that Iran had the highest incidence of sigmoid volvulation secondary to megacolon with an average of 85%, Bolivia 74%, Ethiopia 54%, Pakistan 30%, Russia 30–50%, India 24%, Uganda 20%, Polinia 17%, and the United States 5–10% [4]. On the other hand, the incidence of intestinal volvulus, regardless of the cause and origin, represents variable ranges according to the statistics available; it is reported as 4% of all cases of intestinal obstruction in developed countries and up to 50% of developing countries. Regarding gender distribution, it has been proposed that the predisposition of men to sigmoid colon volvulations is secondary to the fact that the female pelvis has more space for spontaneous reduction of volvulations [7]. A study conducted in the endemic population of Peru showed that fluctuations in temporary rains condition variations in the chances of infection in domestic and human animals [10].

4. Pathophysiology

The vector transmission cycle of Chagas disease begins with the suction of blood from infected mammals by hematophagous vectors, in which the Trypanosome develops until it reaches the infectious phase that is excreted through feces, with which inoculation occurs when feeding on other mammals again by means of mucous membranes or skin lesions that are produced during scratching or bites of the same insects [11]. According to the form of infection and the age at which the infection develops, Chagas disease can present at the level of intrauterine development (10% of positive serologies in childhood and adolescence), having a significant variation in prevalence according to the area and country studied, where up to 81% of pregnant women with Chagas disease have been reported in rural areas of South American countries [12] with varying degrees of morbidity in fetal development and birth, such as abortion, prematurity, low birth weight, and clinical picture ranging from asymptomatic patients to those who develop sepsis, as well as hepatosplenomegaly, meningoencephalitis, hepatitis, myocarditis, and hemolytic anemia [9], although there are also reports of pregnant patients with an acute period of the disease in whom there is no transmission of the parasite to the embryo nonfetus, with which it is determined that the condition can be placental without affecting the fetus, or the fetus without affecting the placenta or generating no affection to either of them despite having an acute period of the disease in the pregnant woman [5].

T. cruzi reaches fetal circulation by hematogenous route as a result of placental inflammation, causing acute or chronic inflammatory foci with parasitism in trophoblastic and macrophage cells, without having a direct correlation between parasitism and fetal infection, since approximately 70–80% of cases despite infection at birth no specific symptoms are found.

When the infection is acquired by vector, it has an incubation period of approximately 5–14 days after direct contact of the parasite with the host when it is by direct inoculation and 20–40 days when it is carried out through blood transfusions [11]. But regardless of the route of infection, Chagas disease has three well-defined stages of development:

- Acute phase: it is usually asymptomatic and presentation in young people, when signs and symptoms occur they are usually transient and coincide with periods of high parasitemia that normally lasts for 2–4 months [1], 1–2% of cases in patients are determined at this stage. When symptoms occur, these are usually frequent and irregular fever that usually extends from 2 to 4 weeks, edema, satellite lymph nodes, hepatomegaly (approximately 40% of cases), splenomegaly, anorexia, asthenia, myalgia, headache, and occasionally arthralgia, [12] and to a lesser extent, data of acute myocarditis (weak pulse, tachycardia, hypotension, cyanosis, edema, and anasarca) [1].

  During this period, you can find signs of entry, also known as "inoculation chagomas," which consist of skin lesions in sites exposed to the vector that have an average duration of 15 days. The most characteristic sign of this period is the so-called "Sign of Romagna—Mazza," which consists of unilateral eyelid edema, pink-light violet, painless, and hard (**Figure 1**) [12] that disappear in an average of 30–60 days [1]. In general, the acute stage develops with a benign evolution, being only fatal between 2 and 7% of cases [12], when it occurs in children under 6 years of age where virulence is greater and they develop lethal meningoencephalitis in 50% of cases [1].

- Chronic indeterminate or latent period represents 50–70% of patients with Chagas disease and is characterized by specific symptoms at the cardiac or digestive level; patients have positive serology and immunoglobulin G for Chagas; however, the rest of the paraclinical studies are negative. About 30% of patients persist with this indeterminate form during the rest of their lives, and the rest evolves to the determined phase in a period of 10–30 years [11]. During this period, you can find indeterminate electrocardiographic manifestations (arrhythmias or tachycardia) and may cause sudden death in sporadic cases.

- Chronic period determined: the parasites have caused damage mainly in tissues of the autonomic nervous system and striated muscles [1]; for this reason, patients have specific organic conditions at the cardiac, esophageal, and colonic levels (among others), in which organomegalies with functional conditions are present, there may be involvement of several organs in the same period. At this stage of the disease, there is a high parasitemia and antibodies. At this point, specific organic conditions allow the use of specific imaging and laboratory studies that favor diagnostic suspicion [12]. Cardiac injuries condition the establishment of chronic Chagasic cardiomyopathy and esophageal symptoms such as dysphagia, odynophagia, hypersalivation, belching, heartburn, and regurgitation, while at the colonic level, they present constipation, meteorism [1], elongations, mesenteritis retractable, and in more advanced cases, intestinal occlusion secondary to intestinal volvulations.

Once the parasite comes into contact with a host cell, it adheres to the specific receptors of the cell membrane and subsequently conditions a restructuring of the microfilaments of the wall, also causing an abnormal mobilization in the calcium channels [1].

In those known as mega syndromes, the megaesophagus and the Chagasic megacolon stand out (**Figures 2** and **3**). The first usually occurs before age 40 and

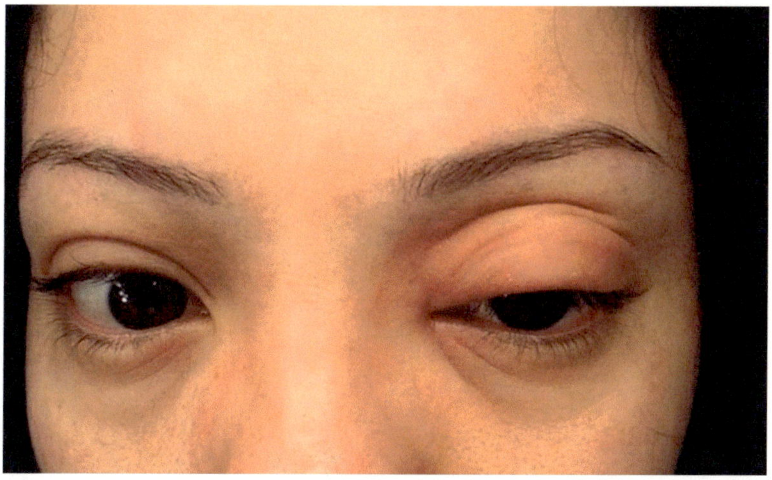

Figure 1.
"Sign of Romagna—Mazza", unilateral eyelid edema, pink-light violet, painless and hard.

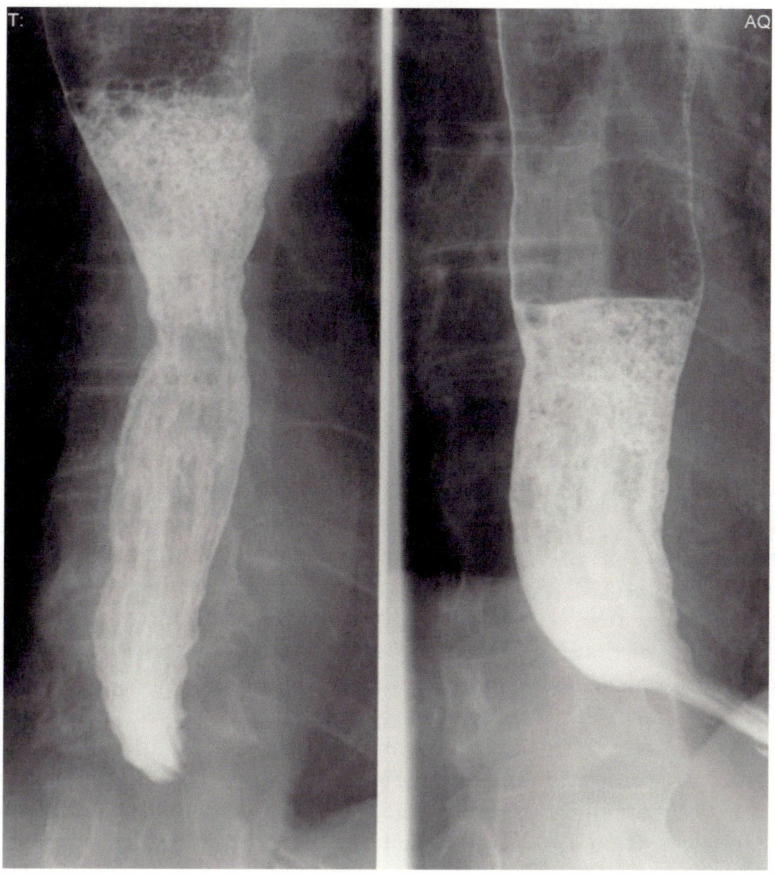

Figure 2.
Contrasted radiography of Chagasic megaesophagus.

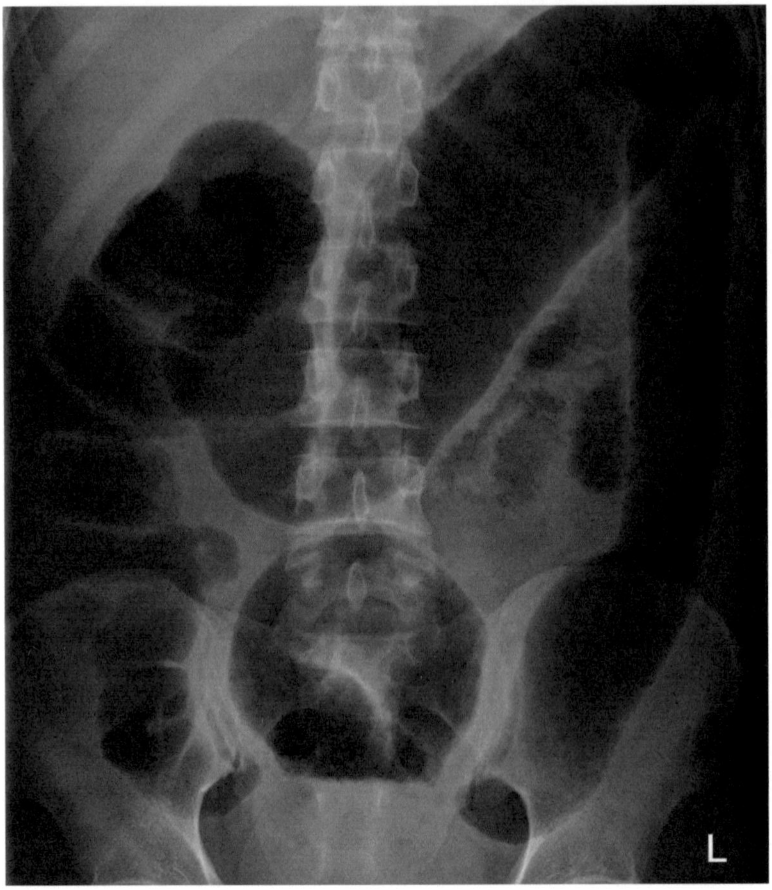

Figure 3.
Simple radiography with dilated colon due megacolon.

is related to the progressive destruction of parasympathetic neurons, which cause dilation in different degrees and subsequent elongation, with hypertrophy of the muscular layers and mucous parakeratosis, with areas of chronic inflammation, which progresses to the progressive loss of motor coordination and contractile capacity, producing dysphagia as the main symptom.

The megacolon usually presents with motor dysfunction of different segments of the colon, being greater in sigmoid and rectum, conditioned by intramural parasympathetic denervation, progressively leading to dilation, presenting as the main complication of it, the development of intestinal volvulations with secondary intestinal obstruction [12]. Another of the factors that are considered associated is the retractable mesocolitis, which predisposes the retraction of the distal and proximal segment of the sigmoid loop favoring its torsion, the copious intake of fermentable and high cellulose foods is also considered a trigger for intestinal volvulations, because with this the elastogenesis is reduced, with elongation of muscle fibers that favors the development of greater volume and length of the handles, since they condition the elongation of the axes in formation of new fibers, it is also considered that the altitude in the inhabited areas could condition a progressive elongation of the intestinal handles according to the physical law of Boyle and Mariotte favoring the expansion of intraluminal gases at a lower atmospheric pressure [4], which is demonstrated from multiple studies in those found that altitude conditioned a significant increase in colonic length in patients living in mountain areas of different countries, proposing the added classification of megacolon height.

From the genesis of the megacolon, it has been classified as congenital megacolon (as an example Hirschsprung's disease) and the acquired megacolon (which includes that caused by American trypanosomiasis) [3], indicating that the volvulations they have are within their etiological factors, the deficit of vitamins, intoxications, and adherent syndromes by chronic or recurrent inflammatory processes [2].

Some authors mention that, in general terms, it can be considered that two essential factors are required for the development of sigmoid volvulus:

1. Redundant segment of colon with a short mesentery.

2. A fixation segment with short proximity to the intestinal loop [3].

The colonic loop conditions the gas and fluid distention of the proximal segment, resulting in a progressive increase in intraluminal pressure that leads to the obstruction of venous return with a congestive picture and finally compromised blood flow of the affected segment, which in If not resolved, conditions ischemia, necrosis and subsequent intestinal perforation.

It is estimated that approximately 40–60% of patients who present with acute abdominal symptoms have previously presented occlusive and distention conditions [13]. In any case, the pathophysiological understanding of intestinal volvulations continues to be poor [14], due in part to the large percentage that is presented urgently with acute abdomen, which is complex, determining the factors prior to such presentation.

5. Clinical presentation

Clinically, sigmoid volvulus may present acutely with surgical resolution, which may present a high rate of complications with morbidity and added mortality in cases where gangrene occurs or when the patient has significant systemic comorbidities [15], or chronic with intermittent and isolated periods of constipation or occlusion that remits spontaneously, many times without reaching the diagnosis of megacolon or volvulation by resolution without treatment [7].

The clinical picture of Chagas disease will depend, as mentioned above, on the clinical phase or stage that is being studied in the patient at the time of the appearance of symptoms. However, making an approach to the development of megacolon (normally observed between 40 and 50 years of age), which leads to intestinal obstruction, by progressive and chronic intramural denervation of the parasympathetic system, it can be mentioned that in a large part of the cases it presents with nonspecific symptoms such as progressive constipation and inability to evacuate, developing intermittent symptoms of generalized abdominal distention, which is usually treated by the patients themselves with laxatives and enemas, which delays medical evaluation and timely diagnosis [12].

The acute clinical picture occurs in approximately 80% of patients [7] and is characterized by sudden abdominal pain and inability to channel gas and stool deposition, conditioning a progressive distention of the abdomen, which in some cases can be asymmetric [10] secondary to the accumulation of gas, fluid, and inflammatory bowel process due to occlusion [3], which increases morbidity [7] and mortality, which can be estimated at 33–80% in cases where intestinal ischemia occurs [16], which can lead to necrosis in three areas mainly in the neck of the volvulus, at any location of the occluded closed loop, and in the portions adjacent to the volvulated area (distal descending colon or proximal rectum by venous thrombosis backward) [6]. Mortality also rises considerably in those with decompensated systemic comorbidities [17]. In a study conducted in India, with a sample of 128 cases of patients with sigmoid volvulus, it was found that 93.75% presented what was considered a classic clinical triad that included abdominal pain, distention, and constipation [7]. According to the time of evolution, the patient may have aggregate symptoms such as nausea and vomiting of gastrointestinal characteristics [18], as well as tachycardia, hypotension, and polypnea, due to the development of systemic inflammatory response syndrome.

Volvulations, unlike fecal impaction, condition an empty rectal ampulla, and the distention is usually more intense than obstructions at higher levels of the gastrointestinal tract [6]. If the picture is not resolved, the patient will present data from peritonitis secondary to necrosis of the intestinal walls, which can lead to perforation of the hollow viscera with the intestinal contents leaving the peritoneal cavity.

6. Diagnostic methods

Depending on the clinical stage of Chagas disease, the level of blood parasitemia, detection, and isolation of *T. cruzi* may be relatively easy; in the neonatal period, for patients who are at risk of vertical transmission from an infected mother, obtaining umbilical cord blood is the method of choice [1].

Direct methods for the isolation of the causative agent can be performed with fresh examination, thick drop, Strout's concentration method (blood collection without anticoagulant for centrifugation of red blood cells and leukocytes not trapped in the clot), triple centrifugation, and microhematocrit [2]. Indirect methods are based on the study of the patient's immune response and are mainly used in chronic phases when the number of parasites in the blood is less than the acute phase; it is considered that there must be two positive tests taken in the same blood sample and include at least one of the tests considered to be the most sensitive (ELISA or indirect immunofluorescence), in case of discrepancies, a third test or referral to a laboratory would be performed specialized [19].

For the specific case of the Chagasic megacolon and the sigmoid volvulus, the diagnosis is initially based on extensive history, including housing history, work areas, chronic digestive symptoms, and the time of establishment of acute intestinal occlusion symptoms [7]. On physical examination, data related to intestinal obstruction will be revealed, including generalized abdominal distension, peristaltic noise fighting with metallic sounds [17], generalized tympanism, and abdominal pain that may or may not have frank data of diffuse peritonitis.

The clinical picture of intestinal obstruction, vomiting, distention, abdominal pain, and chronic constipation accompanied by X-rays constitutes the basic pillars for diagnosis [14]. Simple abdominal radiography reaches diagnostic percentages greater than 90% [20], where you can find the classic sign of volvulations with coffee bean or omega image [18] (**Figure 4**), which is observed in approximately 30% of the cases [14], as well as classic signs of secondary occlusive conditions and

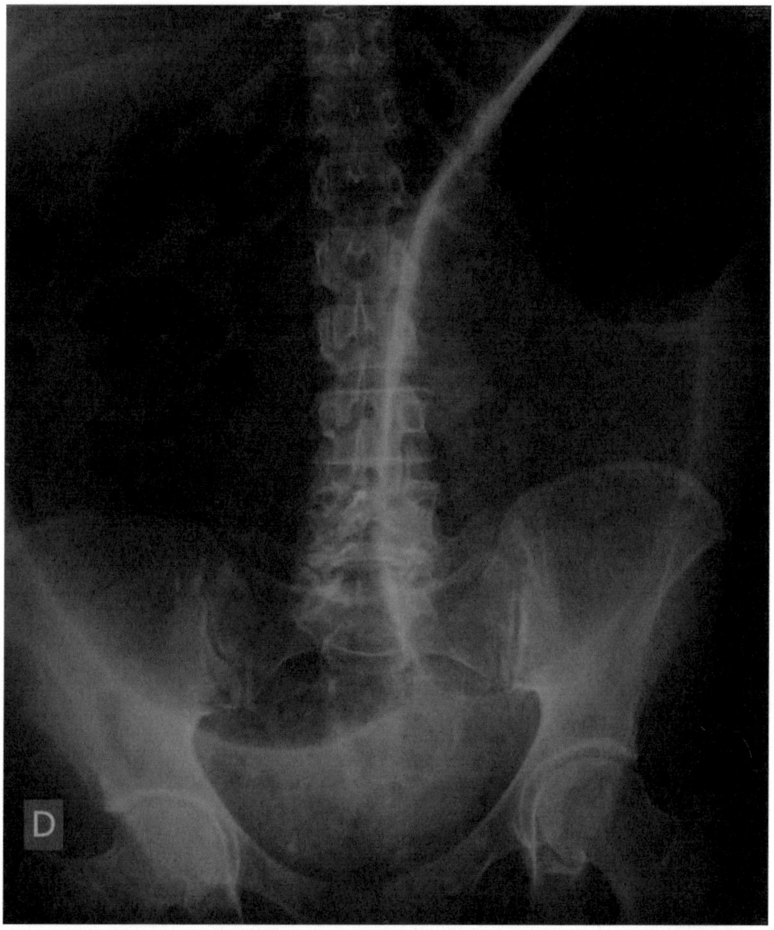

Figure 4.
Coffee bean imagen in simple radiography due sigmoid volvulus.

other pathologies such as coin stack, hydro levels, inverted "u", etc. [20] (**Figure 5**). In cases where the diagnosis is not established with the aforementioned, the use of studies contrasted with barium by enema may show obstruction at the level of the rectosigmoid junction with a bird's beak image, so that the diagnostic method can approach the 100% [6]; it is also considered that this type of studies can have a therapeutic purpose generated a detortion in many cases [14]; however, its use is limited due to the risks of peritonitis perforation and development, in which it is contraindicated [18]. The tomographic study can reveal the classic image of swirl sign due to the rotation of the mesocolic vessels turned (**Figure 6**), also having the advantage of ruling out other abdominal pathologies that occur with similar symptoms [16].

Despite the fact that the clinical picture and imaging tests allow the diagnosis to be elucidated in most cases, there are still variable percentages in which the diagnosis is established intraoperatively after starting the procedure under the approach of the acute abdomen or intestinal occlusion (**Figure 7**) [17].

Endoscopic studies such as rectosigmoidoscopy and colonoscopy make it possible to have a diagnostic-therapeutic possibility in patients with sigmoid volvulations while providing the ease of making an internal evaluation that helps predict the possibility of intestinal ischemia [20].

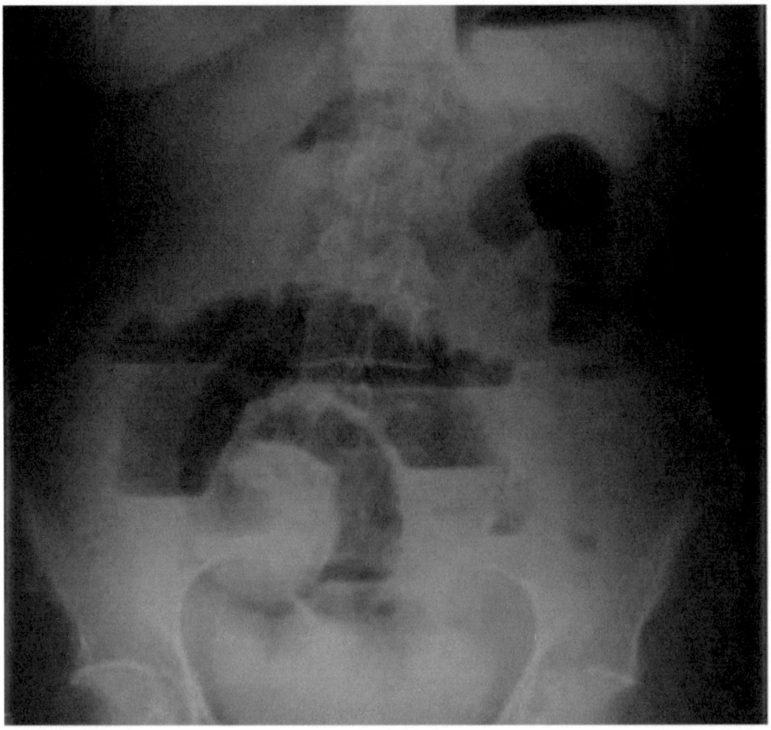

Figure 5.
Simple radiography with coin stack, hydro levels and inverted "u" imagen.

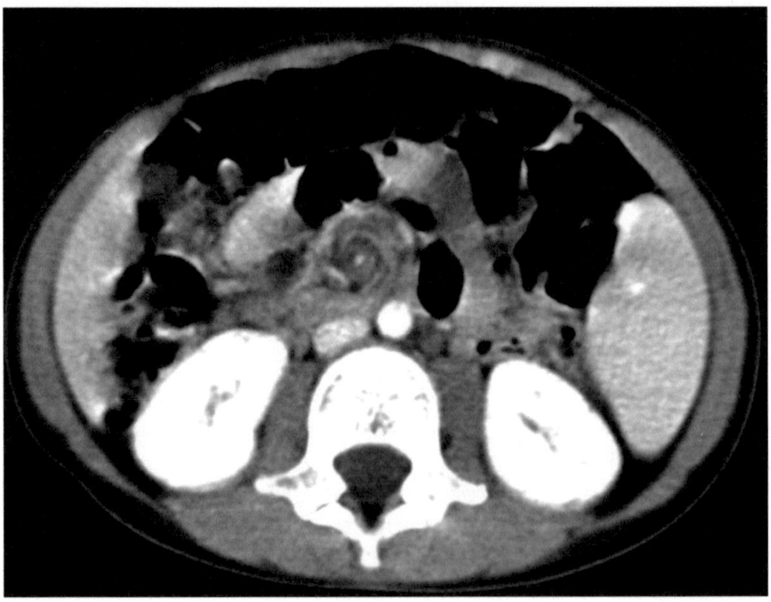

Figure 6.
Swirl sign due to the rotation of the mesocolic vessels.

Among the differential diagnoses that should be ruled out are stenosant colon neoplasms, diverticular disease, pseudo colonic obstruction (Ogilvie syndrome), megacolon due to Hirschsprung's disease, and other intestinal tract volvulations [13].

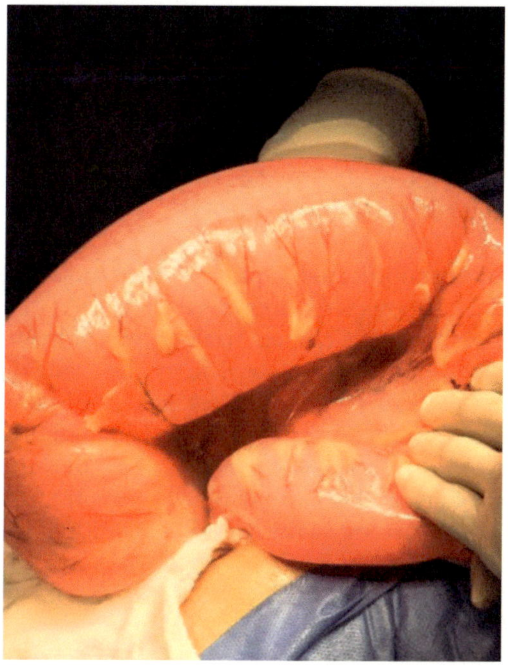

Figure 7.
Intraoperatively finding of sigmoid volvulus.

7. Treatment

The specific treatment of Chagas disease continues to be a challenge and health concern in countries that are considered endemic [1], and throughout history, different drugs have been used for their management, finding useful specific Nifurtimox and Benznidazol, which act on the circulating form of *T. cruzi*, so the best healing results are obtained when administered in the acute phase of the disease [2]; however, its use in pregnant patients is restricted by the risk of teratogenicity [1]. In case of patients who have acquired the disease vertically, the efficacy of the etiological treatment is estimated to be close to 100% in the first year of life, demonstrating elimination of parasitemia and negativization of serological tests within a few months of starting the treatment [21]. Approved treatments for etiological management are not commercialized on a daily basis, and their use depends on the national health agencies of each country. The recommended intake duration for treatment is 60 days, although in cases where there are adverse reactions that cause intolerance, a shortened therapy of 30 days can be considered, subsequently completing the other 30 days with the unused medicine once adverse effects have been controlled [19].

Different treatment schemes have been proposed according to the patient's age, but in general terms, the doses proposed and analyzed as effective in parasite eradication are follows:

- Benznidazole: 5–10 mg/kg/day divided into two daily doses for 60 days and may vary up to 7 mg/kg/day with the recommendation to be administered after food to reduce the risk of adverse reactions, which include dermal hypersensitivity, generalized edema, fever, myalgia, arthralgia, nausea, vomiting, hyporexia, anorexia, epigastralgia, leukopenia, thrombocytopenia, agranulocytosis, and purpura.

- Nifurtimox: 10–15 mg/kg/day in two daily doses for 60 days with the recommendation of being administered after food and performing a weight control at each assessment to identify the need to adjust the dose. Among the side effects or adverse reactions that have been reported are abdominal pain, epigastralgia, anorexia, weight loss, vomiting, instability in balance, confusion, seizures, chills, memory disorders, mood swings, insomnia, nervousness, rashes, generalized edema, and pruritus [1].

This medication is contraindicated in patients with moderate to severe hepatic, renal, or neurological conditions with immunocompromise.

So far there are no comparative clinical trials between the two drugs approved for etiological treatment, so the use will depend on the availability of the drug and the patient's tolerance to it [21]. The cure criterion is the obtaining of two negative samples for parasitological and serological study consecutively at intervals of 6 months after the end of the pharmacological treatment [1]. In cases where the patient is in the intermediate and chronic stages, the treatment is mainly based on resolving the symptoms according to the specific organic conditions that occur (heart disease, megaesophagus, megacolon, etc.), [11] such as diuretics, beta blockers, angiotensin converting enzyme inhibitors [19], possibility of pacemakers, or even considering the requirement of heart transplantation. The management in case of esophageal conditions is based on the use of endoscopic dilations, [11] application of botulinum toxin, and so on.

As mentioned earlier, sigmoid volvulus is considered an emergency for management; however, the pathophysiological characteristics of those that are secondary to Chagasic megacolon have percentages with spontaneous resolution before vascular complications develop in the mesentery of the affected loop. There is no general consensus about the surgical treatment of the Chagasic megacolon, since in some cases, the expectant or conservative management is reserved for patients in whom the symptoms are mild and intermittent and have a functionality compensated with dietary management or with judicious use of laxatives, as well as in those patients in whom comorbidities result in a surgical contraindication. It is important to mention that the surgical management of the Chagasic megacolon does not lead to the cure of Chagas disease, since at the time of presentation of these complications, patients usually present organic dysfunctions at different levels, so they are out of etiological treatment; however, megacolon management favors the resolution of constipation symptoms and reduces the risk of acute complications such as sigmoid volvulus or fecalomas [22].

Among the most frequently used elective procedures are:

- Rectosigmoidectomy: used since 1955, it can be performed with primary anastomosis or colostomy bypass and subsequent anastomosis; however, high rates of stenosis and fistulas have been reported.

- Anterior rectosigmoidectomy: it does not imply perineal affection; allows a variable resection of the affected segments; allows to manage a single surgical time with less morbidity, thanks to the use of mechanical sutures; and does not generate manipulation of the sphincter complex.

- Duhamel Haddad technique: it consists of resection of the affected segment with proximal colostomy and preservation of the native rectum, and it is used by surgeons with experience in colorectal approaches, so its use by surgeons with little experience leads to a higher rate of complications.

- Habr-Gama and Reis Neto procedure: allows a surgical time with mechanical sutures in which adequate morphological results are obtained, functional while maintaining the observation of the patient [22].

When the presentation of the megacolon is performed with intestinal volvulations, the treatment must be aimed at the resolution of the obstruction and prevention of recurrent episodes [13]; however, the treatment remains controversial, and the procedure of choice is based on the general condition of the patient, the suspicion of peritonitis, the viability of the volvulated segment, and the experience of the surgical team [14]. Therefore, the treatment can be divided into two main branches: emergency surgical management and conservative (nonsurgical) management [16].

- Conservative management: in many places, the initial procedure of choice is considered, since it allows decompression and resolves the acute problem, which allows planning a definitive procedure electively reducing the risks of urgent surgery [23]. This approach in deferred times has been widely accepted as the standard management [7]. Conservative procedures include the following:

    - Endoscopic unwrapping: it is indicated in the initial stages, when there are still no vascular damages in the volvulated loop. The basis of this treatment is the decompression by evacuation of the proximal intraluminal content and elimination of pathological rotation of the colonic mesentery [3]. The importance of endoscopic evaluation is based on the intrinsic observation of the volvulated handle and consists of the insertion of a rigid or flexible rectosigmoidoscope that allows the application of air and resolution of volvulus with a success rate ranging from 70 to 90% [13]; however, these procedures have a high risk of perforation. In any case, laparotomy should be performed in all cases where endoscopic findings show necrosis, mucosal ulceration, or inadvertent intestinal damage [17].

    - Sigmoidopexy and mesosigmoidoplasty have a low morbidity and mortality rate; however, they have a high incidence of recurrences [7] (**Figure 8**).

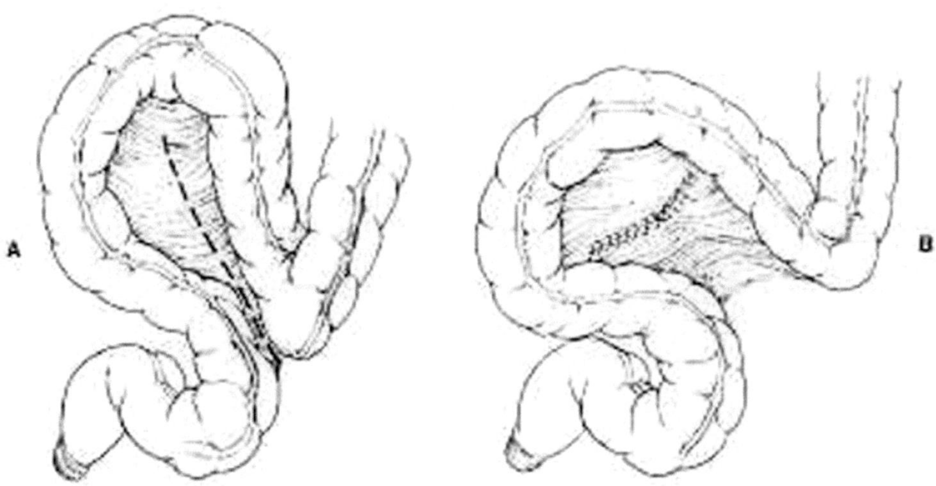

Figure 8.
Mesosigmoidoplasty technique. (A) Incision of relaxation on the longitudinal mesentery. (B) Transverse mesentery closure.

- The colon by enema has shown a success rate close to 5% of patients, with a lower recurrence rate in pediatric patients [13], while providing a diagnostic confirmation; however, it is contraindicated in patients in whom ischemia or intestinal necrosis is suspected due to the risk of perforation.

Conservative procedures are considered an effective measure for the resolution of the emergency; however, they must be completed with elective surgery given the high rates of recurrence they present, in addition to many of the patients in which they are performed, do not return to units for surgical complementation until they have an acute condition again [20].

- Surgical management: emergency laparotomy is indicated in those patients in whom clinical signs suggest ischemia, necrosis, or intestinal gangrene (leukocytosis, fever, vomiting, severe abdominal pain, data of peritoneal irritation, hypotension, free air in abdominal cavity, acidosis, or frank sepsis data) [16]. The patient's clinical status, transoperative findings, the presence or absence of peritonitis, and the preference of the surgical team are what will determine the management of the volvulus [18]. Among the therapeutic options are in the following:

    - Colopexia: it is performed in cases where the surgical examination shows intestinal viability, without data of ischemia or necrosis, and consists in the reduction of the volvulate loop and subsequently fixing it to the abdominal wall in order to reduce the risk of recurrence, with a lower mortality rate [24].

    - Intestinal resection with primary anastomosis: the surgical procedure of choice is currently considered in patients in whom ischemia of the proximal and distal areas is not observed, after resection [7]; however, this procedure is even in controversy due to the lack of preparation of the colon in emergency surgery and the risk of dehiscence of the anastomosis [13], which is estimated at an approximate percentage of 5.5% [18].

    - Intestinal resection with Paul-Mickulicz technique: it consists of resection of the volvulated segment that includes the mesenteric neck, which in many cases requires a wide mobilization of the rectum to perform externalization of the proximal and distal loop, which is complex to perform in patients undergoing emergency surgery [7].

    - Intestinal resection with Hartmann technique: resection of the volvulated segment with closure of the distal loop and externalization of proximal colostomy is indicated in those patients in whom ischemia of the proximal and/or distal intestinal segments is observed, or intestinal gangrene with data of peritonitis, as well as in those in whom the primary anastomosis is considered at high risk of leakage due to the preoperative state of the patient [7].

8. Conclusion

Megacolon, as a complication in the chronic stage of American Trypanosomiasis or Chagas disease, is a frequent cause of intestinal obstruction secondary to dilated loop volvulation in countries where the disease is considered endemic.

In countries that are not considered endemic, consensus has been proposed for early detection in primary health systems, since a lack of information has been detected in professionals at this level of care [25]. The detection of biochemical markers allows to generate a long-term correlation of the risk of cardiomyopathy and mega syndromes associated with parasitemia levels [26]. Treatment in the acute stage of the disease leads to a high cure rate; however, many of the patients do not receive timely treatment due to nonspecific symptoms in this period. The treatment of the volvulations will depend on the clinical state of the patient, being able to opt for management with or without intestinal resection of the first instance, through endoscopic approaches or emergency surgery. For patients with any sign of peritoneal irritation who are judged as already suffering bowel gangrene, emergency operation must be attempted. Because urgent approaches under general anesthesia have shown a higher rate of postoperative complications, models of minilaparotomy under regional anesthesia are positioned as another therapeutic option in high-risk patients for emergency surgery [27]. By contrast, for clinically stable patients, that is, those with no signs of peritoneal irritation, endoscopic reduction is the first acute care option of choice and has been widely accepted with a high success rate and low morbidity and mortality rates [28]. However, this is only a temporizing procedure, and a high recurrence rate has been reported. Therefore, it is strongly recommended that endoscopic reduction should be followed by elective definitive surgery that is recommended to perform laparoscopically with primary anastomosis [29]. There are studies in which the approach with local anesthesia for intestinal resection has been proposed in patients with uncomplicated volvulations and low-risk patients, as an alternative for the definitive management of this disease [30]. For cases in which the surgical risk due to comorbidities contraindicates surgery, procedures with assisted colopexia and percutaneous colostomy have been shown to have good results for relapse prevention [31]. Similarly, the use of simple percutaneous endoscopic colostomy with a probe has also proven to be efficient in elderly patients [32]. Monitoring through *T. cruzi* urinary antigens has proven to be an efficient method for the detection of Chagas disease reactivation in patients presenting with HIV coinfection [33]. The clinical signs and the general condition of the patient will condition the basis for the final management of intestinal obstruction; however, the etiological cause of the volvulation should be monitored.

Author details

Víctor Hugo García Orozco
Hospital Civil de Tepic "Dr. Antonio Gonzalez Guevara", Tepic, Nayarit, México

*Address all correspondence to: victor-garcia.cirugia@hotmail.com

References

[1] Paredes R. Prevalencia de chagas congénito en recién nacidos del "Hospital Materno Infantil Poconas". En: Ramos M, Serrudo J, editores. Ciencias de la Salud T-I Handbook. Bolivia: ECORFAN; 2014. pp. 189-218

[2] Mansilla M, Rocha M, Sarubbi M. Chagas congénito. Presentación de un caso clínico y revisión bibliográfica. Revista del Hospital Materno Infantil Ramón. Sardá. 1999;**18**(1):29-35

[3] Frisancho O. Dolicomegacolon Andino y vólvulos intestinales de altura. Revista de Gastroenterología del Perú. 2008;**28**:248-257

[4] Saravia Burgos J, Acosta CA. Megacolon y vólvulo de sigmoides: Incidencia y fisiopatología. Revista de Gastroenterología del Perú. 2015;**35**(1):38-44

[5] Moya P, Basso B, Moretti E. Enfermedad de Chagas congénita. Aspectos epidemiológicos, clínicos, diagnósticos y terapéuticos. Experiencia de 30 años de seguimiento. Revista da Sociedade Brasileira de Medicina Tropical. 2005;**38**(Suppl 11):33-40

[6] Hellinger MD, Steinhagen RM. Colonic volvulus. In: Wolf BG et al., editors. The ASCRS Textbook of Colon and Recta Surgery. New York, NY: Springer; 2007

[7] Janardhana Rao K, Podili NK, Rajagopal M. Review of sigmoid volvulus: A 5 years experience in tertiary care hospital, Visakhapatnam. Journal of Evidence Based Medicine and Healthcare. 2018;**5**(25):1948-1953. DOI: 10.18410/jebmh/2018/405

[8] Secretaria de Salud. Prevención y Control de la Enfermedad de Chagas, Programa Sectorial de Salud 2013-2018. México, D.F: Secretaria de Salud; 2014

[9] Freilij H, Altcheh J. Congenital Chagas disease: Diagnostic and clinical aspects. Clinical Infectious Diseases. 1995;**21**:551-555

[10] Levy MZ et al. Bottlenecks in domestic animal populations can facilitate the emergence of *Trypanosoma cruzi*, the aetiological agent of Chagas disease. Proceedings of the Royal Society B. 2015;**82**:20142807

[11] Enfermedad de Chagas. The Center for Food Security & Public Health. Institute for International Cooperation in Animal Biologics; 2009

[12] Werner Apt B, Heitmann I, Jercic M, Jofré L, Muñoz P, Noemí I, et al. Enfermedad de Chagas en el adulto, la infancia y la adolescencia. Revista Chilena de Infectología. 2008;**25**(3):194-199

[13] Rodríguez U, Badillo A, Cruz J, Rovelo E. Vólvulo de sigmoides en el Hospital Juárez de México: 20 años de experiencia. Revista Mexicana de Coloproctología. 2006;**12**(3):112-116

[14] Mulas C, Bruna M, García-Armengol J, Roig JV. Management of colonic volvulus. Experience in 75 patients. Revista Española de Enfermedades Digestivas. 2010;**102**:239-248

[15] Irsulla V, Ojeda LA. Vólvulo del sigmoide en la enfermedad de Chagas. MEDISAN. 2011;**15**(7):1014

[16] Katsikogiannis N, Machairiotis N, Zarogoudilis P, et al. Management of sigmoid volvulus avoiding sigmoid resection. Case Reports in Gastroenterology. 2012;**6**:293-299. DOI: 10.1159/000339216

[17] Turan M, Sen M, Karadayı K, Koyuncu A, Topcu O, Yıldırır C, et al. Our igmoid colon volvulus experience

and benefits of colonoscope in detortion process. Revista Espanola de Enfermedades Digestivas. 2004;**96**:32-35

[18] López J, Tallon L, Sánchez L, López J, Mompelan O. Tratamiento del vólvulo de colon sigmoide mediante detorsión endoscópica seguida de sigmoidectomía asistida por laparoscopia en régimen de urgencia diferida. Case Reports in Gastroenterology. 2012;**6**:293-299. DOI: 10.1159/000339216

[19] Salazar P, Bucio M, Cabrera M, De Alba M, Castillo D, et al. Enfermedad de Chagas en México. Revista de la Facultad de la UNAM. 2016;**59**:3

[20] Khanna A. Sigmoid volvulus: A nonresective alternative for viable sigmoid colon. JIMSA. 2012;**25**:1

[21] Cucunubá Z, Valencia C, Puerta C, Sosa S, Torrico F, Cortés J, et al. Primer consenso colombiano sobre Chagas congénito y orientación clínica a mujeres en edad fértil con diagnóstico de Chagas. Infection. 2014;**3**:3-16

[22] Santos R, Meyer B, Féres O, Ribeiro J. Surgical treatment of Chagas megacolon. Critical analysis of outcome in operative methods. Acta Cirúrgica Brasileira. 2008;**23**(Suppl 1):83-92

[23] Fry R, Mahmoaud N, Maron D, Ross H, Rombeau J. Colon an rectum. Colonic volvulus. In: Sabiston Textbook. 18th ed. USA: Elsevier; 2008

[24] Rajsiddharth B, Reddy S, Srinivas B, Sriramoju S, et al. A Clinical study of sigmoid volvulus. International journal of Scientific Study. 2016;**3**:10

[25] Saumell C, Soriano A, Solsona L, Gascon J. Documento de consenso sobre el abordaje de la enfermedad de Chagas en atención primaria de salud de áreas no endémicas. Atent Primaria. 2015;**47**(5):308-317

[26] Sabino E, Ribeiro A, Lee T, Oliveira C, Carneori A, et al. Detection of *T. Cruzi* DNA in blood by PCR is associated with Chagas cardiomyopathy and disease severity. European Journal of Heart Failure. 2015;**17**(4):416-423

[27] Ernesto L, Kareem A. Minilaparotomy without general anesthesia for the treatment ofsigmoid volvulus in high-risk patients: A case series of 4 patients. International Journal of Surgery Case Reports. 2017;**34**:23-26

[28] Scharl M, Bierdermann L. A symptomatic coffee bean: Acute sigmoid volvulus. Case Reports in Gastroenterology. 2017;**11**:348-351

[29] Atamanalp SS, Atamanalp RS. Determination of patients requiring elective surgery following successful endoscopic detorsion in sigmoid volvulus. Pakistan Journal of Medical Sciences. 2017;**33**(6):1528-1530. DOI: 10.12669/pjms.336.13921

[30] Tavassoli A, Maddah G, Noorshafiee S, Salehi M, Imannezhad S, et al. Acta Medica Iranica. 2016;**54**(10):640-643

[31] López A et al. Endoscopic treatment of recurrent sigmoid volvulus with colopexy assisted by T-fasteners and colostomy. Endoscopy. 2016;**48**:E236-E237

[32] Frank L et al. PEC for sigmoid volvulus. Endoscopy International Open. 2016;**04**:E737-E741

[33] Castro Y, Gilman R, Mejia C, Clark D, Choi J, et al. Use of a Chagas Urine Nanoparticle Test (Chunap) to correlate with parasitemia levels in T. cruzi/HIV co-infected patients. PLOS Neglected Tropical Diseases. Feb 2016;**10**(2):e0004407. DOI: 10.1371/journal.pntd.0004407